SILENCE & DISSENT
EXPERT DOUBT IN THE AIDS DEBATE

Alan McManus

COPYRIGHT

First published in Scotland, 2017

Copyright © Alan McManus

All rights reserved.

ISBN-13: 978-1981832972

ISBN-10: 1981832971

CONTENTS

THANKS iv
INTRODUCTION 1
HIV AS THE (PROBABLE) CAUSE OF AIDS 14
   A Metaphor for the Perplexed 15
HIV AS A COFACTOR OF AIDS 20
   The HIV Story 22
   Black Correlation 26
   Epidemiology & Etiology 28
ANTI-HIV DRUGS: SIDE EFFECTS & ADHERENCE 34
HIV AS HARMLESS; AIDS AS INCOHERENT 45
   Haemophiliacs 48
   Africans 55
   Gay Men 61
TESTING TESTING 71
   ELISA & Western Blot 72
HIV AS INEXISTENT; AIDS AS INCOHERENT 79
   Straining the Imagination 85
   Strategies of Dissent 89
   Isolation of HIV 93
   T-Cells & Viral Load 97
   Electron Microscopy 99
   Deaths of Dissidents 102
   ART & Liver Failure 106
AFTERWORD & *APOLOGIA* 110
BIBLIOGRAPHY 118
ABOUT THE AUTHOR 122
DEAR READER 122

THANKS

To my beautiful tan terrier Ben, who yawned and moaned and pushed his shaggy head between me and the keyboard when he was bored and felt we both needed to go out for a refreshing walk. Thanks to Dr Christopher Onyiaodike, Dr Sunday Swift and Mr David McFadyen, for very helpful feedback on a succession of drafts. All of these good people bear absolutely no responsibility for the content of this book. Thanks also to Christian George who has released his photo, 'Assorted Condoms', which I have used for the cover of this book, into the Public Domain on: www.publicdomainpictures.net.

To João

Who taught me about antibodies

Gusto muito de você, leonzinho

As what is immature is destined to become mature, what buds to become full-blown (fledglings to become full-fledged) – the doctors' botanical or zoological metaphor makes development or evolution into AIDS the norm, the rule. I am not saying that the metaphor creates the clinical conception, but I am arguing that it does much more than just ratify it. It lends support to an interpretation of the clinical evidence which is far from proved or, yet, provable.

(Susan Sontag, *AIDS and its Metaphors*, p.29)

INTRODUCTION

Standing at the back of the Cathedral (because the pews are packed) I see speaker after speaker who would not otherwise darken the door of a place of worship – and wholeheartedly despise organised religion – ascend the wooden steps of the high pulpit, and I listen to them recount stories of faith and hope and love to the faithful below. At some point, amid the red balloons and festoons of rainbow tape, below the banners proclaiming WE ARE ALL INNOCENT and THERE IS NO DEATH: THERE IS ONLY LIFE, candles are lit, and held up. And there is a reading of names. Amid the silences that follow, we murmur names of the faithful departed, our beloved dead. Our lovers, our kin, our stars, our friends.

We will remember them, but this is no Remembrance Day Service. Three weeks after the eleventh day of the eleventh month, we gather in the evening to remember the dead who bore no arms except their own, who loved and lost their lives against an implacable and inhuman enemy (despite its name). From the going down of the sun and in the morning, we will remember them. Their absence accompanies us though all our daily rituals and even, especially, on our holidays. There are two lines of separation here: one between the quick and the dead; one between the negative and the positive. No, in this instance, it is preferable to be negative.

This is our faith. This is our practice. This World AIDS Day Service, generously supported by large pharmaceutical companies and attended by people who live their lives in the earnest attempt to be the solution: to be open, to be free, to love spontaneously, to give generously, to care for the Earth and all her peoples, to save the whales and to walk their dogs and to be inspired, in a thoroughly disorganised and understated sort of spirituality, by the wonders of Nature, and by the diversity of humankind and by the small acts of kindness that (despite our systems of structural injustice and personal meanness of character) we persist in committing, daily.

The atmosphere is holy, special, set apart. This is time out, time for reflection. They who have gone before us, wherever they have gone, have run out of time. We have not. So we must use our time to best advantage. Because time flies. And for some of us, perhaps many, in this place tonight, time is fleet-footed indeed. All we can do is cherish each other, for the time we have left together, and work for a solution that will extend that time. Until our inhuman enemy, HIV, the slinking emissary of AIDS, is finally defeated.

If it ever existed in the first place. Or if it were ever harmful. Imagine the rage that would course through the pews like a purifying fire, if such thoughts, such criminal and impious thoughts, were ever voiced aloud in such a setting. Imagine the inundation of indignant words against such thoughtcrime, such insensitivity, that would dare to suggest that all this piety, all the docility of those we love (surrendering their bodies to the side-effects of AZT/ ART/ HAART, succumbing finally to PCP, KS and liver failure) all this was mistaken. There is only one word for such impiety: heresy.

Dr Ben Goldacre, a medical doctor, quality newspaper journalist and documentary-maker whose bestseller *Bad Science* was followed by another, *Bad Pharma*, details why we need to take the subject of HIV and AIDS seriously:

> AIDS is the opposite of anecdote. Twenty-five million people have died from it already, three million in the last year alone, and 500,000 of those deaths were children. In South Africa it kills 300,000 people every year; that's eight hundred people every day, or one every two minutes. This one country had 6.3 million people who are HIV positive, including 30 per cent of all pregnant women. There are 1.2 million AIDS orphans under the age of seventeen. Most chillingly of all, this disaster has appeared suddenly, and while we were watching: in 1990, just 1 per cent of adults in South Africa were HIV positive. Then years later, the figure had risen to 25 per cent. (Goldacre/2009/182)[1]

No-one sane and of good-will would argue with Dr Goldacre about the continuing great harm done by HIV/ AIDS phenomena. Experts may argue whether the cause is environmental, virological or iatrogenic (literally 'doctor-caused'), but all agree that too many lives have been ended or ruined in connection with these phenomena. However, Philip E. Johnson, Professor of Law at the

---

[1] Dr Goldacre does not reference his source for these figures on this page but the chapter (published in the 2009 not the first, 2008, edition) refers in its endnotes to pp. 184 & 185 to two studies, both entitled "Estimating the lost benefits of antiretroviral drug use in South Africa", both published in 2008, by N. Natrass in *African Affairs* 107 (427): 157-76 and by P. Chigwedere, G.R. Seage, S. Gruskin, T.H. Lee and M. Essex in the *Journal of Acquired Immune Deficiency Syndromes* (*sic*) 49 (4):410-15, respectively.

University of California, Berkeley, comments on what he terms, "The Thinking Problem in HIV-science":

> The HIV establishment has made much of a 1994 paper by Dean Mulder *et al*, in *Lancet* [vol. 343, p. 1021], titled 'Two-Year HIV-1-Associated Mortality in a Ugandan Rural Population'. This study of Ugandan villagers showed that those who tested positive for antibodies had a much higher death rate than those who did not, especially in the age group 25-34. Officials from the CDC and other AIDS agencies cite this study as proving that an AIDS epidemic caused by HIV is ravaging Africa.
>
> What the HIV propaganda does not say is that the subjects did not die of AIDS. The cause of death was reported for 64 antibody-positive subjects, and of this group *only* 5 were diagnosed as AIDS under the very broad 'Bangui' (African) definition, which requires only conditions like sustained weight loss and persistent diarrhoea. Moreover it is erroneous to assume that the Ugandans who tested positive were actually HIV-infected, because false positives on antibody tests are common, particularly in Africa. That this finding of mostly non-AIDS deaths among persons who may or may not have been HIV-infected was claimed to support the HIV theory of AIDS and the existence of an African HIV/AIDS pandemic is eloquent testimony to the closed mindset and intellectual dishonesty that rules HIV research. (Johnson/1996/335, gloss and emphasis original)

The problem appears to be that the focus of the medical establishment is not on whether research findings are scientific but on whether they are acceptable to the major medical and pharmaceutical stakeholders. Dr Malcolm Kendrick, whose *exposé* of pharmaceutical harm, *The Great Cholesterol Con*, provoked outrage from those who profit from selling statins, details similar attacks on expert authors who dare to question the received wisdom on any treatment from radical mastectomy to mortality rate vs BMI:

> Do I really believe that we are heading for some form of totalitarian state, where dissent against the medical 'experts' will be punishable by imprisonment? Well, yes, I do. We are already in a situation where doctors who fail to follow the dreaded 'guidelines' can be sued, or dragged in front of the General Medical Council, and struck off. Thus losing their job, and income. (Kendrick/2014/129-130)

Both Dr Kendrick and Dr Goldacre underline the importance of medical data to distinguish verifiable fact from anecdote and Professor Johnson the issues of the reliability of such data, and the possibility of researcher bias in either its collection, analysis or subsequent reporting. So the verification of facts and hypotheses on HIV/AIDS is crucial. Complicating a hypothesis to explain collected data and then collecting more data that necessitate complicating it even further is not the same as verifying the facts supposedly supporting a hypothesis. Especially while ignoring the data that contradict it. HIV-AIDS research literature abounds in phrases such as 'surprising', 'puzzling' and 'unexplained'. The confusion goes back to an announcement in 1984 to the press, about a probability. The press published it as a certainty. Subsequent studies – and the published research that followed it, which should have preceded it – have done likewise. But not all. Science also advances by dissent.

There's a surprise in Dr Robert Gallo's book, *Virus Hunting: AIDS, Cancer and the Human Retrovirus*. Not that the title mimics Dr Paul de Kruif's bestseller *Microbe Hunters* or that Dr Gallo makes a series of ungenerous remarks about his French scientific counterpart Dr Luc Montagnier (Gallo/1991/146-176, 212)[2] but that he admits his approach to this research was deductive.

For fans of Sherlock Holmes, the word 'deduction' conjures up images of the great detective on his hands and knees in a lovely lady's boudoir, triumphantly pouncing on a cigarette end and announcing that a swarthy gentleman measuring six feet two and thirteen stones seven (who had eaten kippers for breakfast and arrived at the scene of the crime in a Hansom cab) was the culprit.

For empirical researchers, the word is rather more specific. Research is, typically, approached either inductively or deductively. 'Induction' in this context means the process of letting the analysis of the data lead to the theory. 'Deduction' means the opposite: testing an already constructed theory. Sherlock Holmes tends to use the former, not the latter. Most detectives do. Apart from young, sassy (usually female) Criminology graduates in American cop shows who announce confidently to the older (usually male) officers that the criminal (also usually male) will fit the expected profile.

---

[2] *Virus Hunting* was published in 1991 when Dr Gallo was Chief of the Laboratory of Tumor Cell Biology at the National Institutes of Health in Bethesda, Maryland and Dr Montagnier Chief of the Laboratory of Viral Oncology in the Department of Virology of the Institut Louis Pasteur, Paris.

Dr Gallo (1991/5) says:

> I decided to find out if retroviruses could indeed cause cancer in humans. To do this it would be necessary to find at least one retrovirus that caused cancer in at least some humans.

There's nothing unscientific about a deductive approach to research. Testing a theory is one of the main things that science is supposed to do. As long as the researcher is clear about the criteria required for a theory to pass the test – and honest when a certain theory fails to satisfy them.

The astute reader will, at this point, wonder what approach I'm taking to the writing of this book and what my criteria are for either the construction or the testing of theory. Firstly I will point out that, as a non-scientist whose title of 'Dr' is not medical but refers to my Ph.D. in the philosophy of education, **I am in no position to either test or construct any theory relating to such a grave issue as HIV/AIDS.**

All I can do is to use my skills in scanning complex technical documents and in written communication of key ideas. The first comes from my experience as a proofreader and the second from my own doctoral research as well as my experience of being a teacher and university lecturer. In other words, **no-one should make potentially life-threatening decisions based on my perceived opinion of the contents of this book.**

I am absolutely *not* advising anyone to mistrust medical and scientific authorities. I will, however, point out those instances where medical and scientific authorities – even at the highest level – are in disagreement over whether one side or the other have succeeded in satisfying the accepted empirical criteria for their far-reaching conclusions. This book is written organically to demonstrate the existence of an on-going debate, not systematically to draw that debate to a conclusion, and there is no testing of biomedical theories here. Rather I seek to present the various, conflicting, answers (put forward by competent authorities) to these questions:

1 – Does HIV exist?

2 – Is HIV the cause of AIDS?

The purpose of writing this book is to provide people who have taken, or are thinking of taking, one of the various types of HIV test with some clarity about the range of controversies which have dogged these tests since their invention – and also some clarity about the stated aim and side effects of the various drugs officially recommended for those who test positive to having HIV antibodies. It is wearying to have to scour the internet trying to find clear answers to reasonable questions about risks to one's health only to encounter *ad hominem* attacks, crazy conspiracy theories, pharmaceutical propaganda, racism, homophobia, and the circumlocution and confusion that are the hallmarks of bad science.

The phrase 'competent authorities' is rather vague. Who am I, not a medical doctor nor a scientist, to decide who is competent to present a view on such matters? I, clearly, am incompetent to do so. In this case, I trust to the evaluations of the medical and scientific establishment.

Therefore, for the purpose of this book, 'competent authorities' are those accepted by the medical and scientific establishment as such *even by those in disagreement with them over certain issues concerning HIV/AIDS* and notwithstanding their relationship with other public figures or private bodies – including large pharmaceutical companies.

For example, the well-documented scientific disagreement and political settlement for patent fraud between the HIV researchers Dr Robert Gallo and Dr Luc Montagnier do not contradict their established standing as competent authorities in this field.

As for how I set out to conduct this search for answers, I must admit that there is no statistical analysis of the results of internet and university library keyword searches, with clear exclusion criteria. This is for two reasons: firstly because, as a proofreader, I have waded though pages of postgraduate methodology chapters (typically with plagiarised misunderstanding of the 'research onion' diagram and absolutely no attempt to even *admit* researcher bias, let alone balance it). Believe me, there is nothing so boring. My aim is to write a book that people would actually want to read. People who would rather not read detailed scientific articles but want a general picture.

Secondly, because neither my very limited experience as a voluntary auxiliary nurse in a hospice nor my many years of carework for various client groups qualify me in any way to interpret biomedical findings. Therefore I must trust to the interpretation of competent authorities when explaining these findings for a non-expert readership or audience. I also try not to fatigue the reader – for example, Dr Gallo has a rather jolly writing style whereas Professor Duesberg's detailed prose can be a bit heavy-going.

Now I need to confess my motivation and initial bias. As a man who first had a boyfriend in the 1980s (we didn't use that heteronormative term then, to me he was my lover) HIV and AIDS have always been of great concern. I have three times taken HIV tests, all in Scotland, and all were negative. The last was months ago. I know other people, some in other countries, who have had a positive result (the man to whom this book is dedicated is not one of them).

Obviously, I would not have taken those tests if I had not had some belief in the possibility of the HIV-AIDS link being factual. I am writing this introduction at the beginning of this search for answers and, right now, I would say that I am about 98% sure that this link has never been proved to be factual. I can confidently say, at least, that it has never been proved to my satisfaction.

So what? Who am I to demand scientific certainty when I can't even understand the published proof? Should I not either shut up and meekly accept the findings of those who can – or go off and study for years until I am qualified to understand them for myself?

I already have 5 or 6 degrees (it depend how you count them) and although I have proofread the most complex scientific and medical documents, to Ph.D. level, prepared students for their doctoral *viva* (successfully) and coached medical researchers in presentation skills, I have always been clear that in doing this work my competence is limited to the English language (although some of my work with the medical researchers was in Italian).

So, when Dr Eleni Papadopulos-Eleopulos *et al.* (1997)[3] state that "there is ample evidence that reactions between "HIV" proteins and "HIV" antibodies are non-specific", I cannot argue that these reactions are not. I can hardly even understand what that means. I wouldn't know an 'HIV protein' from an eyelash. All I can do is to see whether, as she claims, other competent authorities state the same thing – and whether this statement confirms or contradicts their other statements. The answers, therefore, must show consensus.

---

[3] "HIV Antibodies: Further Questions and a Plea for Clarification" by Eleni Papadopulos-Eleopulos, Valendar F. Turner, John M. Papadimitiou, Gordon Stewart and David Causer (most of 'the Perth Group') published in *Current Medical Research and Opinions* Vol. 13: 627-634, 1977, available at: http://helpforhiv.com/proteins.htm – posted 2007, accessed October 2017. The Perth Group repeated their statement that such reactions appear non-specific in "HIV – A Virus Like No Other", published & posted 2017, accessed October 2017, available at: http://theperthgroup.com/HIV/TPGVirusLikeNoOther.pdf

In 2017, at least in post-industrialised countries, it's commonplace that patients demand to be able to make informed choices, as much as possible, about their care. Women no longer simply submit to the demands of (male) obstetricians that they should be supine, shaved, drugged, panicked, and that their newborn should be subjected to the harsh glare of lights, loud noise and instant cord-cutting. There is information about these things, there are choices.[4] People who have cancer are encouraged to use whatever complimentary therapies that ease the impact of radiation and chemotherapy side effects on their bodies.[5]

The days of 'shut up we know what's best for you' are over. Or should be. People who have cancer don't need to see the electron microscope evidence for their particular strain in order to make good, informed, decisions about their diet and exercise regimes. Expectant mothers who couldn't explain the difference between DNA and RNA (or care less about it) can still make the right choices about soft lighting and quiet to ease their baby into the world.

Clearly the situation with HIV is different. The difference is that, to my knowledge (and I know many people who have had cancer and many mothers) no competent authority is currently questioning the existence of cancer or saying that women give birth better without any assistance at all.[6]

---

[4] See: www.positivebirthmovement.org/

[5] See: www.maggiescentres.org/

It is not surprising that people receiving devastating news want to have as much clarity as possible about it. Questions raised about HIV, its existence, its identity and its causative relationship with AIDS (itself a medical anomaly if there ever was one) have apparently, in 2017, still not been adequately answered.

I say 'apparently'. This book is written in the realization that the big picture of these questions and answers is lost in the details. Meanwhile, people are taking life-threatening decisions in ignorance of other biomedical points of view. It is commonplace nowadays to say that 'HIV+ people' and 'people with AIDS' are 'living longer'. But if people are still dying and if competent authorities are still arguing why – is it not a moral imperative for all of us (patients, care-givers, support staff, loved ones, politicians, celebrities, clergy, biomedical researchers, concerned fellow human beings, alike) to admit to what extent we are in fact living with ignorance, trying to distinguish reality from illusion in a hall of mirrors?

---

[6] Although, given the reported bullying by some male obstetricians, I believe there is a certain feeling that way!

HIV AS THE (PROBABLE) CAUSE OF AIDS

Dr Robert Gallo, in giving the background to his published article following the famous press release by Margaret Heckler, US Secretary of Health and Human Services, in April 1984,[7] describes "the presence of a virus-specific enzyme" (reverse transcriptase or RT) as "a way around the problems of electron microscopy" – which included the fact that he did not have such a microscope in his lab (all Gallo/1991/70-71). In this description there is a telling sentence:

> To the extent that the test for the viral form of the enzyme could be made both sensitive and specific, I would have, in effect, at least a preliminary test for the presence of a human retrovirus. I might still want to confirm my results with an electron microscope, but I would have a basic test, easily performed in my own lab, to begin looking for evidence of human retroviruses. This became my long-term objective. (Gallo/1991/71)

This objective was in the context of the large-scale funding of the American 'War on Cancer' supported by the US President:

> The National Cancer Act was passed in 1971 and signed at a large press conference by Richard Nixon two days before Christmas. Some lobbyists had openly boasted this would bring about a cure for cancer by 1976. Others drew the analogy with the moon landing, persuading

---

[7] Part of the controversy over the Secretary's announcement was that: "In 1983, Dr Luc Montagnier [claimed to have] discovered the virus that causes AIDS, which he called LAV. He sent his findings to Dr Robert Gallo [...] to have him examine them. Although what exactly transpired still remains debateable, Dr Gallo maintains that he independently discovered the AIDS virus, which he named HTLV-III, in 1984." (Feldman & Wang Miller/1998/15, gloss & ellipsis mine).

legislators that the shower of money would work similar miracles for medicine. (Duesberg & Ellison/1996/104)

With all this public money being poured into biomedical research, and all this publicity, researchers were under pressure not only to prove that a human retrovirus existed but that it caused cancer. However, when Dr Gallo shared his work with colleagues in the Virus Cancer Program at their annual meeting in Hershey Pennsylvania, it attracted derision:

> As the time of the meeting approached, our own follow-up studies started to suggest what we had earlier failed to consider: the possibility that the retrovirus we were finding was a contaminant, or contaminants, of animal retroviruses also being studied in our laboratory. (Gallo/1991/84)

In the late 1970s, funding was cut:

> The Virus Cancer Program left its special mark on biomedical research. [...] The message was clear [...] decisions about the direction and funding of biomedical research can suddenly become very political, and woe unto any scientist who finds himself [sic] in the field of fire. (Gallo/1991/92, gloss & ellipsis mine)

A Metaphor for the Perplexed

Before we go any further, it may be helpful to explain some of the biomedical vocabulary that has already been used and prepare ourselves for even more. Sometimes I find it helpful to have a kind of very vivid metaphor, 'mind-map' or 'theatre of memory' of iconic elements, in my mind to understand something intricate. Please remember that this metaphor is entirely of my own invention and therefore is both inadequate and a gross oversimplification of the complex theories of virology.

Let's imagine a cell, human or animal, as an office. There are all sorts of things in this office, some of them may be deadly, sometimes a dividing wall appears, sometimes a bit of the office takes itself off somewhere else, sometimes two offices combine…so the metaphor as a whole is clearly faulty but each iconic element functions as a place-holder for a biomedical feature of HIV. Let's just concentrate on two aspects: the manager and the secretary.

Just for the sake of making the metaphor more memorable, let's imagine a typical American 1950s office (as least as portrayed in sitcoms) where a Mr Moody is the boss and Lucy the secretary. Now the boss (the DNA) has a clear role: to direct operations in the office (the cell). He does this by expressing himself (gene expression) and the secretary (the RNA) takes her cue from him. Not so in this office! Because Lucy acts like a retrovirus. Not only does she originate from outside (let's say Lucy was a client of Mr Moody's bank) but when she manages to get herself into the office she turns everything on its head because it's not the boss calling the shots, it's Lucy!

So a retrovirus propagates when its RNA invades a cell and programs the DNA of that cell to make more of this virus. We can think of a retrovirus as an uppity (or empowered) secretary. If this image is annoying you, that's good. It will stick better in your mind.

Remember you're only reading this because you can't be bothered ploughing through biomedical documents, so put up with it!

Reverse transcriptase (RT) is the enzyme that makes this process possible.[8] Let's imagine that Lucy has a very alluring perfume that Mr Moody can't resist and that this is the secret of her power grab. (I know this is outrageous, just go with it.) Even if Lucy (retroviral RNA) wasn't observed in the office (host cell), the presence of the perfume (RT enzyme) would be enough to alert an observer to her activity there.

Or would it?

We haven't covered all the necessary vocabulary yet, so let's add more details to this office (cell) scenario. Lucy (retroviral RNA) also has a large bunch of keys (surface glycoprotein 120 knobs) that she uses to open office doors using the keyhole (CD4 receptor site). Lucy also has stiletto heels (transmembrane gp41), a bulging handbag (capsid protein24) and permanently permed hair that's actually a wig (matrix p17). What are they in our running metaphor? Proteins, of various densities. Of course, Lucy isn't the only lady to have those kind of heels or that brand of handbag, the contents of which are generic – for example, a lipstick (integrase p32) and a powder puff (nucleocapsid p7(9) – and the RT (p66) perfume can be

---

[8] "RNA-based viruses (**retroviruses**, as they are known) have a special enzyme, a **reverse transcriptase**, which copies their own message into a DNA segment. This is inserted into their host's DNA, which is forced to make many copies of the RNA retrovirus." (Jones & Van Loon/2001/110, emphasis original).

in the handbag too).⁹ Lucy also has pepper spray (protease p12) handy, just in case.

Now, imagine that the observer who was trying to ascertain whether Lucy (retrovirus) was present (or had ever been present) in the office (cell) was both deaf and blind. No problem: there's the giveaway presence of her perfume (RT enzyme). But what if this observer didn't have a great sense of smell? What if the office (cell) had geraniums growing in pots on the windowsill, a lavender essential oil plug-in behind Lucy's desk and a coffee machine that was permanently switched on behind Mr Moody's? What are all these? Distractions. Cellular debris.

What I do know is that the simple presence of a strong smell in the office doesn't necessarily mean that it's the smell of perfume. It certainly doesn't mean that it's necessarily the smell of Lucy's perfume – as there may be other secretaries wandering in and out of the office and what about Mr Moody's *Eau-de-Cologne* and what about Mrs Moody?

---

[9] I realize that this cartoon version of Lucy the retrovirus is structurally unsound – as the surface knobs sit on top of the transmembrane protein, that puts her keys on top of her stiletto heels! But you get the picture. Nomenclature of proteins and glycoproteins is from "Morphogenesis, Maturation and Fine Structure of Lentiviruses" by Hans. R. Gelderblom *et al.* (1990/160). There is a *tenuous* link between the elements of the office and of the invaded cell (e.g. the capsid, that contains other viral proteins, being a handbag; and protease, that defends against viruses, being pepper spray) but the important point is the illustration of the difference between a 'characteristic' and a 'specific' quality of a retrovirus/ HIV.

I know I'm having fun with this, but this is the serious point that Dr Papadopulos-Eleopulos and her research colleagues of the Perth Group have been making for decades when they question whether reactions between 'HIV proteins' and 'HIV antibodies' have been proven to be specific. Rather than simply characteristic.

It may be *characteristic* of Lucy's perfume (RT enzyme) to be strong-smelling, but it's certainly not specific. Because there are lots of strong-smelling things in that office which are not that perfume. This is why it was so important for Dr Gallo that "the test for the viral form of the enzyme could be made both sensitive and specific" (Gallo/1991/71). Despite official assurances to the contrary, as recently as July this year (2017) the Perth Group stated that Dr Gallo's hastily patented HIV test was neither.[10]

---

[10] See "HIV – A Virus Like No Other", published & posted July 2017, accessed October 2017, available at:
http://theperthgroup.com/HIV/TPGVirusLikeNoOther.pdf

HIV AS A COFACTOR OF AIDS

Working at a Retreat Centre one Christmas, I printed out all the relevant verses from the synoptic gospels (Matthew, Mark, Luke) and asked the guests to arrange them in a coherent order, to tell the story of the nativity of Jesus. Everyone knew this story and could repeat chunks of it off by heart, 'there were shepherds, tending their sheep', 'no room at the inn', 'laid in a manger', 'gold, frankincense and myrrh', etc. Except that when we tried to put all the various accounts together, we found that they didn't fit.

It is widely accepted among Liberal Christians that scripture contains many instances of 'a story to tell a truth'. This phenomenon of meaningful but perhaps not totally factual narratives is not limited to religion. In Scotland right now we have the *Time for Inclusive Education* campaign to get LGBT education into schools. I wrote a booklet for them (McManus/2013) to help with the special problem of getting into Roman Catholic Schools. Recently, one of the key supporters of this campaign tweeted that 'gay liberation started at Stonewall'. This young man is in his 20's and is Scottish. In making this statement he ignored all the indigenous patrons of homosexual rights in these islands, as diverse in time and nature as the flamboyant wit Oscar Wilde, more than a century ago, and the furtive Joe Orton whose documentary *Prick Up Your Ears* portrayed 'cottaging' in a time of criminalisation, decades before the famous riots at the Stonewall Bar in New York's Greenwich Village, in June 1969. And even those events are disputed.

Volunteering at a stall (for a gay-friendly Episcopalian church) at Glasgow Pride a couple of years ago, I got chatting with someone I presumed was either transvestite or transsexual. I didn't spend time trying to work out which, because it was none of my business but I was quite prepared for the word 'transgender' to come up in the conversation. Especially since we happened to be talking about Stonewall. I was therefore surprised when this person punched the air on informing me that, "it wasn't the trannies who led the charge against the police at Stonewall, it was the lesbians". (Yes, it's an in-group word also used as an insult by those outside.) I realised two things simultaneously: firstly, this person – who appeared to be genetically male – was most likely either intersex or, post-transition, no-longer identified as transgender but as simply a woman and (being attracted to women) as lesbian. Secondly, grand narratives have a life of their own.

The phrase 'grand narratives' comes from *The Postmodern Condition: A Report of Knowledge* by Jean-François Lyotard (1979) and refers to story-telling as the means not only of the propagation of knowledge but of its legitimisation.[11] Science is full of examples and many are quite charming. Archimedes in his bath discovering mass, Newton under the apple tree discovering gravity, Kekulé dreaming

---

[11] See: www.marxists.org/glossary/terms/g/r.htm

of a snake swallowing its tail and discovering the cyclic structure of benzene. Just because the story may not prove to be factual doesn't mean there is no truth in the knowledge the story imparts.

The HIV Story

Samuel V. Duh (M.D., M.P.H.)[12] takes up the idea of narrative:

> So the story goes like this: There is a close similarity between STLV-III (SIV) and HTLV-III (HIV); SIV is isolated in African green monkeys, and the green monkeys have close contacts with humans in Central and East Africa; the cross-reaction between SIV and HIV is more common to Africans. Therefore, SIV got into humans in Central and East Africa. [...]
>
> The speculation is that the green monkeys bit humans and transmitted SIV. Alternatively, humans ate green monkeys with SIV infection and thus contracted the virus. SIV underwent mutation to become HIV and somehow maintained a silent infectious state. During the immediate postindependence years (the early 1960s), many of the countries in Central and East Africa required expert knowledge; the experts who came included Haitians. The Haitian experts (mostly men) had sex with African women who were infected with HIV. They returned to Haiti and spread the virus in heterosexual and bisexual populations. Homosexuals from San Francisco went to Haiti on vacation, had sex with infected bisexuals, and contracted the virus. [...] some of the

---

[12] John H. Stanfield II, College of William and Mary, Editor of the Sage Series on Race and Ethnic Relations, describes Dr Duh as: "a physician with extensive clinical and research experience on AIDS" (Duh/1991/vii).

> European experts also had sex with infected African women and similarly introduced the virus to the homosexual population in Europe. The virus spread from homosexual IV drug users to heterosexual IV drug users, and then it finally spread to the rest of the population. (Duh/1991/61-62, ellipsis mine. IV = intravenous)

The above paragraphs are from Dr Duh's book, *Blacks and Aids: Causes and Origins*. He has the following reflections on this story:

> The story as I have narrated above has been the "official" scenario of the origins of AIDS/HIV infection. I have heard officials from the CDC give this scenario. I have heard officials of state public health departments give the same scenario. And I have heard infectious disease specialists, recognized in their communities as AIDS experts, give the scenario. The story is told so matter-of-factly that there seems to be no doubt about it. But the story of where HIV originated and how it spread is just that – a *story*. (Duh/1991/62, emphasis original)

I, for reasons previously stated, can't be the judge of whether this story is true or not. But it does seem rather complicated. Dr Duh wrote this version of the HIV/AIDS origin story in 1991. Sixteen years later, researchers at the University of Arizona published their findings:

> Monkey viruses related to HIV may have swept across Africa more recently than previously thought, according to research from the University of Arizona in Tucson. A new family tree for African green monkeys shows that simian immunodeficiency virus first infected those monkeys after the lineage split into four species. The

new research reveals the split happened about 3 million years ago. Scientists had thought SIV infected an ancestor of green monkeys before the speciation event.

"Studying SIV helps us learn more about HIV," said the paper's first author Joel Wertheim, a doctoral candidate in the UA department of ecology and evolutionary biology. [...]

["]All SIVs and HIVs have a common ancestor["], added senior author Michael Worobey, a UA assistant professor of ecology and evolutionary biology.

[...] Green monkeys almost never get sick from SIVagm. If SIVagm was once a monkey killer, the change in its virulence may shed light on the future course and timing of the evolution of HIV.[13]

I'm interested in these findings for three reasons. Firstly, before Dr Montagnier's international lawsuit against Dr Gallo's patent was quashed diplomatically (Presidents Chirac and Reagan had to intervene to prevent embarrassment)[14] Dr Gallo called his 'AIDS virus' HTLV-III. Which, purely in terms of nomenclature, is STLV-III (SIV) with the H for 'human' substituting the S for 'simian' (monkey).

Secondly, Dr Gallo reported that the ridicule he experienced at the annual meeting of the Virus Cancer Program was not personal but professional:

---

[13] www.sciencedaily.com/releases/2007/07/070716132633.htm – posted 2007, accessed October 2017, gloss and ellipsis mine.

[14] Dr Gallo (1991/205-216) relates the entire (official US) story.

> Several researchers, one after another after another, came up to announce that the examination of the cells we had sent out for independent confirmation had revealed not one, but two – and in the case of one cell line, three – different animal primate retrovirus combinations. (Gallo/1991/85)[15]

On the same page, a footnote reveals that this contamination was widespread in laboratories:

> Oddly enough, after the evidence that our isolate was a monkey virus, several groups in Europe and at least one in the United States (Werner Kirsten's group at the University of Chicago) reported isolations of the same type of monkey virus from human cells that were, I assume, also contaminants. (*ibid*)

This does give the impression that we shouldn't imagine SIV researchers such as Wertheim and Worobey as intrepid explorers who spend their time up trees in Africa *interacting* with monkeys – but rather as emotionally detached white-coated scientists, living comfortably in post-industrialised countries, who arrange for the capture, breeding and eventual torture of these poor beasts in their well-equipped labs. Dr Gallo does mention one intrepid journalist:

> Amazingly, in the early part of my research on AIDS (early 1983) I was visited by Ann Guidicci Fettner, a freelance writer who told me emphatically that the origins and epicentre of the epidemic were in a river basin near Lake Victoria. She also stated that she

---

[15] The reported contaminants were: "woolly monkey virus, gibbon ape leukemia virus, and baboon endogenous virus" (Gallo/1991/86).

believed the virus came from African green monkeys, apparently due to her experiences and observations in Central Africa. (Gallo/1991/227, footnote)

What is amazing to me is why Dr Gallo, an empirical scientist, even mentions this anecdotal evidence from a journalist intent on a story, no matter how emphatically related nor how strong her belief in her own 'experiences and observations'. It's hard to understand how a medical journalist, notebook in hand, would be given the credence that should be reserved for a trained epidemiologist.

Thirdly, the event that Wertheim and Worobey reported as 'recent' happened at some point in the last 3 million years. And all this is supposed to explain the following statement:

> Citing some laboratory research that suggests HIVs from the late 1980s are more virulent than HIVs from the 2000s, Worobey added, "For HIV, the really cool thing is that these changes can take place on a more rapid timeline that previously thought."[16]

Black Correlation

Dr Duh (whose otherwise informative book, like Dr Gallo's quoted above, tends to conflate HIV and AIDS) notes that: "being black is a risk on its own of acquiring the disease" (Duh/1991/80).[17] This extraordinary statement is quickly qualified:

---

[16] www.sciencedaily.com/releases/2007/07/070716132633.htm – posted 2007, accessed October 2017.

> there is no conclusive evidence that blacks are genetically susceptible to AIDS. Indeed is it questionable that blacks are truly more susceptible. They do not have the highest number of AIDS cases; they do have a *disproportionately high rate* based on their population. If they are more susceptible, I contend that there is an environmental rather than a genetic susceptibility. (*ibid*, emphasis original)

Dr Duh (1991/21) explains this environmental susceptibility in terms of the socioeconomic characteristics of Black Americans:

> black Americans on the average are less healthy than other racial groups. They have relatively lower life expectancy. They have higher mortality rates. Infant health, child and adolescent health, and adult health are all relatively poorer for them. They have high excess death rates and high relative risk rates for most health conditions. They are less likely to be involved in health promotion and disease prevention activities.
>
> Black Americans are on the average also poorer. They are less educated and less employed. Many poor blacks live in crowded housing conditions, where crime, illicit drug use, and prostitution are common. They tend to be uninsured or underinsured. They tend to see doctors less often; they tend to wait until later stages of an illness before seeing a doctor. They tend to use public clinics or hospital emergency rooms instead of doctor's offices.

Dr Duh's explanation centres on the ease of access to the bloodstream:

---

[17] Samuel V. Duh (M.D., M.P.H.) at the time of his writing was Medical Executive Director of the Flagler County Health Department in Florida, after working for the Bureau of Epidemiology, Texas Department of Health, and went on to become the CARE International HIV/AIDS and Health Advisor for Ghana, Togo, and Benin.

And there is nothing inherent in certain racial groups that promotes transmission. Racial differences in AIDS/HIV-infection prevalence have to do with relative efficiency of access to people's blood by HIV. (Duh/1991/34)

Duh sees this access as facilitated by the greater tendency among poor people to have STDs – which result in genital lesions – and to share needles (if they are intravenous drug users).

Epidemiology & Etiology

South African biomedical researcher, Dr Joseph Sonnabend, provides in the first issue (in 1983) of his journal, *AIDS Research*, what could be an alternative explanation for at least some of the homosexual and heterosexual transmission of 'the AIDS virus':

> Entitled "The Etiology of AIDS," the article officially proposed what he called the "multifactorial model" of causation. According to this notion, many different infections could have a combined effect that eventually destroys the immune system. He also hypothesized that semen itself – coming in contact with blood when rectal tissues were torn during anal intercourse – might cause immune suppression. (Duesberg & Ellison/1996/221)

Gordon T. Stewart, Emeritus Professor of Public Health at the University of Glasgow, shares at least some of the conclusions of Dr Duh and Dr Sonnabend on co-factors of the spread of HIV and of progression to AIDS – taking issue with both the orthodox hypothesis of the virus "that HIV is the unique cause of AIDS" (Stewart/1994/168) and the conceptualisation of the syndrome:

> AIDS is registered internationally as if it were a single infectious disease, and is surveyed accordingly, that is to say as if it were a self-defining dependent variable. (Stewart/1994/169-170)

Firstly, rather that the virus being the sole cause, Professor Stewart is in agreement with Professor Duesberg in regard to the alternative explanation that high levels of STIs and drug abuse are, *at least*, co-factors of AIDS:

> The first cases were registered in San Francisco on July 1st, 1981. By March 1985, 1,000 cases had been registered, of which 992 (99%) were male and 98% homosexual or bisexual with multiple partners, with a very high prevalence of gonorrhoea, syphilis, hepatitis and other sexually-transmissible infections, with 13% using intravenous drugs and 98% resident in the Bay area. The position in 1992, in the UK, most of Europe, Australasia and North American at least, is that AIDS is still predominantly a disease of men (Stewart/1994/168-169)

The last point is important to Professor Stewart and other researchers he cites who all emphasize the greater chance of contact between blood and semen in anal sexual intercourse, especially when forceful, and speaks of this chance increasing in some situations: "with 'fisting' and other accessory, traumatic and contaminating procedures, and with multiplicity of partners" (Stewart/1994/176). The mention of the majority residence in the San Francisco Bay area is a reference, for Professor Stewart, to homosexual transmission of HIV facilitated by semen-blood contact.

Although this explanation may appear not to differ at all from the orthodox position, Professor Stewart's conclusion is that HIV is not necessary and sufficient for the development of AIDS:

> AIDS and AIDS-related complexes (ARCS) develop, *with and without HIV*, because heterologous antigens in spermatozoa enter the rectum and bloodstream, or in whole blood and blood concentrates given as transfusions, provoke allogenic responses and elicit antibodies which are toxic to lymphocyctes, and cause a fall in CD4 counts. (Stewart/1994/179, emphasis mine)

I am left to wonder why the HIV hypothesis is necessary at all, if other factors can just as well explain the presenting conditions. Professor Stewart notes that this explanation accounts best for AIDS in 'the Western world', and not elsewhere:

> In Africa, the Caribbean and Asia, notifications of seropositivity to HIV and of AIDS to the WHO [World Health Organisation] are increasing sharply. The epidemiological and clinical patterns, at face value, are different from those of the western world. Cases are reported with equal frequency in males and females and homosexuality and use of drugs are uncommon as risk factors. In place of the opportunistic infections reported in developed countries, tuberculosis, diarrhoeal diseases, malnutrition, exhaustion and early death are the main clinical features. (Stewart/1994/169, gloss mine)

Robert S. Root-Bernstein, Professor of Physiology at Michigan State University, agrees with Professor Stewart in regard to the lack of coherence in the concept of AIDS as a global syndrome and points out the different periods of time in each risk group for progression to AIDS. Professor Root-Bernstein feels that this lack of coherence comes from the failure of many researchers to "examine all of the available studies" or to pay "attention to sophisticated mathematical models of epidemics". He continues this explanation:

> Most hemophilia studies differentiate between hemophiliacs age 25-44 and those over the age of 44, because the rate of AIDS development in the over 44 group is two or four times faster [...] Furthermore, reference to a large body of studies [...] reveals a rate of progression to AIDS among hemophiliacs less than 25 years of age [...] with a slope different than that for homosexual and hemophiliac men in general (all, Root-Bernstein/1994/186)

This is an answer to the first of Professor Root-Bernstein's "Five myths about AIDS that have misdirected research and treatment", from an article of the same title. The second is to the widespread notion that seroreversion (changing from HIV+ to HIV-) never occurs – especially after "infection was demonstrated by isolation of proviral DNA in addition to ELISA and Western Blot methods":

> In fact, several dozen well-documented cases of seroreversion, often accompanied by return to PCR-negative status, have been published. (both, Root-Bernstein/1994/190)

Professor Root-Bernstein's answer to the third myth takes a pop at Professor Duesberg's assertion, "that antibody against HIV is protective", as well as at "those who believe that HIV accounts for all of the immune suppressions in AIDS". This answer relies on results from the PCR method, itself highly problematic (see below):

> a significant proportion of people repeatedly exposed to HIV become PCR positive but remain antibody negative and healthy. Other people repeatedly exposed to HIV remain antibody negative, are PCR negative, but demonstrate T-cell activation towards HIV antigens [...] In short, HIV is controlled by the T-cell response (all, Root-Bernstein/1994/192)

His answer to the fourth myth, ("The only way to treat AIDS is to treat HIV") is no less controversial:

> The evidence that cofactors are necessary to the progression of AIDS has now convinced a number of investigators that no comprehensive treatment of AIDS will be possible without addressing the full range of cofactors that may influence disease progression. (Root-Bernstein/1994/194,195)

His answer to the fifth ("AIDS must have a single etiological agent") is linked to that of the fourth:

> First, there is no documented case of anyone who has developed AIDS who does not have several of the following immunosuppressive agents at work prior to, concomitant with, or following their HIV infection: multiple, concurrent infections with identified immunosuppressive viruses and bacteria (e.g. herpes viruses, hepatitis viruses, and mycoplasmas); immunologic exposure to alloantigens (e.g., semen, blood or lymphocyctes); chronic or high dose treatments with antibiotics; anaesthetics; chronic or high dose use of immunosuppressive addictive drugs irrespective of mode of use (e.g. heroine); malnutrition; and autoimmunity

directed at T-cells subsets […] Second, and conversely, there is no evidence that HIV can cause disease in an immunologically healthy person free of these causes of immune suppression (Root-Bernstein/1994/200)

So there may be more than one explanation for the environmental susceptibility that Dr Duh finds in Black people to HIV/AIDS. Other competent authorities find that there is a similar environmental (toxicological) susceptibility – to 'AIDS related diseases' – in gay men. The questions that remain are: whether such a susceptibility is a cofactor or the sole factor in the production of such diseases; whether such diseases have anything at all in common; and whether HIV itself is still a cofactor in their production or the virus is simply a "harmless passenger" (Duesberg & Ellison/1996/215) if it even exists at all! These questions are explored in the following chapters.

ANTI-HIV DRUGS: SIDE EFFECTS & ADHERENCE

Healthline claims to be "the fastest growing consumer health information site – with 65 million monthly visitors" and reassures us that "Healthline's mission is to be your most trusted ally in your pursuit of health and well-being." So I can imagine that it's the kind of website that anyone who is computer-savvy and has just had an HIV antibodies test come back positive might consult. Especially perhaps, the article, "Antiretroviral HIV Drugs: Side Effects and Adherence" – which has the following, hardly reassuring, paragraph:

> HIV drugs have improved over the years, and serious side effects are less likely than they used to be. However, HIV drugs can still cause side effects. Some are mild. Others are more severe or even life-threatening. A side effect can also get worse the longer you take the drug.[18]

Dr Gallo admits that toxicity is a problem of antiretrovirals:

> The earliest investigations designed to find effective drugs against HIV were with RT inhibitors. The first was with a compound called suramin. [...] Although the laboratory results were impressive and showed some margin of safety (they blocked the virus at concentrations that did not show toxic effects on cells), the clinical studies proved that the drug was too toxic to be safely used. (Gallo/1991/304, ellipsis mine)

---

[18] www.healthline.com/health/hiv-aids/antiretroviral-drugs-side-effects-adherence#overview1 – "Medically Reviewed by Alan Carter, PharmD on June 16, 2016 – Written by Stephanie Watson", accessed October 2017.

However, Dr Gallo is enthusiastic about DNA terminators zidovudine (AZT), dideoxyinosine (ddI) and dideoxycytidine (ddC):

> AZT is another story. It is a powerful inhibitor of the reverse transcriptase step in HIV replication. […] the claims for *some* clinical effectiveness were made only after careful pharmacological studies were completed and after clinical tests showed significant differences in survival and morbidity (incidence of disease) between placebo-treated and AZT-treated AIDS patients. (Gallo/1991/305, emphasis original, ellipsis mine)

> AZT stimulated studies of related compounds [...] which, like AZT, probably work by chain termination. Some that show promise are dideoxyinosine (ddI) and dideoxycytidine (ddC). (Gallo/1991/306, ellipsis mine)

Steve Jones, Professor of Genetics at University College London, explains that there are "only four units in DNA – Adenine, Guanine, Cytosine and Thymine (A, G, C and T for short)" (Jones & Van Loon/2001/53) and that A pairs with T, as G pairs with C (Jones & Van Loon/2001/58). Dr Gallo explains the action of AZT (substituting Thymine) and other such analogues, with the analogy of "a pearl necklace" – and adds a prophetic (unheeded) warning:

> AZT is a pearl without the second hook. It attaches to the growing DNA chain, but it cannot accept the next nucleotide. Thus it is called a *chain terminator*. Of course, our cells make DNA before they divide, and they need enzymes (DNA polymerases) to catalyze this reaction which, although different from viral RT, is related to it in several aspects. AZT therefore, will also have side effects, like most drugs. (Gallo/1991/305, emphasis original)

Dr Gerald Corbitt picks his words carefully but notes the toxicity of AZT, especially to the most vulnerable:

> There is a lack of information about the effects of Zidovudine treatment in women and the drug is not recommended for women who are pregnant. (Corbitt/2001/37)[19]

Dr Corbitt goes on to write on the infamous Concorde study, which certainly showed up significant differences in survival and morbidity even in people without AIDS:

> On a more controversial note, the results of a large Anglo-French three-year study (Concorde) of the effects of Zidovudine indicate that there is no long-term benefit on either survival or progression to AIDS when the drug is given early in the course of infection compared with being given at the onset of HIV disease. (Corbitt/2001/37-38)

As Dr Corbitt sometimes has difficulty with clarity ('early' and 'onset' being difficult for the lay person to distinguish) I quote another source:

> The largest single study of zidovudine monotherapy in asymptomatic HIV infection, known as Concorde, suggested that there was no advantage in starting zidovudine before symptoms develop in the longer term. Almost 1750 participants were randomly assigned either to start taking 1000mg zidovudine a day in four doses, or

---

[19] Dr Corbitt was Consultant Clinical Scientist and Deputy Clinical Manager in Microbiology and Virology at Manchester Royal Infirmary, and Honorary Lecturer in Virology at the University of Manchester, at the time of his writing.

to receive a placebo until they developed symptoms or until they chose to switch from trial capsules to open zidovudine because of falling CD4 cell counts. The results showed that after three years there was no detectable difference between immediate versus deferred use of zidovudine in terms of disease progression, development of AIDS or survival, but that the patients treated immediately had more severe side-effects. [...]

A meta-analysis of 15 of these trials by the HIV Trialists' Collaborative Group published in 1999 confirmed these controversial findings of the Concorde Study – that zidovudine does not increase a person's chances of AIDS-free survival in the long-term, although it does reduce rates of disease progression in the short-term.[20]

Dr Malcolm Kendrick, General Practitioner, educator and web designer for the European Society for Cardiology and the National Institute for Clinical Excellence in the UK, comments on the outcome:

> I have to admit that this trial was far from perfect, as it was not a placebo-controlled study. It was a study of early vs. late treatment. But it does strongly suggest that the sooner you took AZT, the more likely you were to die early, despite the fact that this disease 'markers' were greatly improved.
>
> All of which means that, when you get down to basics, we have one horribly flawed study suggesting AZT may be much better than placebo. We have another, far larger

---

[20] *NAM AIDSMAP*, under "Resources", "HIV Treatments Directory", "Effectiveness", available at: www.aidsmap.com/Effectiveness/page/1730905 – no date, accessed October 2017, ellipsis mine.

> and better controlled study, suggesting early AZT treatment may be much worse than late AZT treatment. Which may be another way of demonstrating that AZT is far more harmful than placebo. Where does this leave us? In a very difficult place. If AZT was, and remains, worse for AIDS sufferers than doing nothing, how could we now establish this? Well we can't.
>
> Equally, how can we know that the newer drugs, and drug regimes, actually work? Well, we can't, because no-one will ever do a placebo controlled study ever again. We only know that the newer drugs are far better than AZT, which, of course, might have been killing people. (Kendrick/2014/193)

So, anti-HIV drugs are now less likely to kill you. If you're in luck, especially at first, the side-effects might only be severe. Some years down the line, you may not be that lucky. From what we now know about the under-reporting of adverse effects,[21] the chances of side-effects of anti-HIV being only 'mild' seem very slim indeed. Let's imagine Joe Bloggs, whose world has just fallen apart, being told to be bodypositive and to thank whatever stars he looks up to that things ain't what they used to be in anti-HIV medicine. What side-effects might he expect? *Healthline* tells us that he'll be on more than one antiretroviral drug for, hopefully, a long time:

> Today, more than 20 antiretroviral drugs are approved to treat HIV. Most people who treat their HIV will take two or more of these drugs each day for the rest of their lives.

With a warning:

---

[21] See *Bad Pharma* (Goldacre/2012) *in toto*.

> Sticking to your treatment plan isn't always easy. These drugs can cause side effects that can be severe enough to make some people stop taking them.

The writer then lists each side-effect, with the "drugs that cause it", and some helpful advice on alleviating it. I've summarised this information in two lists as my purpose is different from that of the writer. She wants to help people feel better while taking these drugs; I want to show clearly that all of these drugs have severe side-effects – that only get worse as time goes on.

The symptoms listed are: Appetite loss, Bleeding, Body fat loss/ gain, Bone loss, Diarrhoea, Fatigue, Fever, Heart disease, High blood sugar/ diabetes, High cholesterol/ lipids, High lactic acid in blood, Insomnia, Kidney damage, Liver damage, Mood changes/ depression/ anxiety, Nausea/ vomiting, Nerve problems (numbness/ pain/ burning in hands/ feet), Pancreatic damage, Rash.[22]

Other sites, such as *HIV InSite*, from the University of California San Francisco, add as many symptoms again.[23] *Healthline*

---

[22] Order, abbreviation/ editing – such as "Body fat loss/gain" for "Lipodystrophy (changes in the distribution of body fat)" – and (UK) spelling are mine. See www.healthline.com/health/hiv-aids/antiretroviral-drugs-side-effects-adherence#overview1 – "Medically Reviewed by Alan Carter, PharmD on June 16, 2016 – Written by Stephanie Watson", accessed October 2017.

[23] Such as: Abnormal dreams, Alopecia, Anemia, Asthenia, Cysts, Dry mouth, Elevated serum creatinine, Fanconi syndrome, Flatulence, Hepatitis, Hyperbilirubinemia, Hyperpigmentation of palms & soles, Hyperuricemia, Intercranial haemorrhage, Jaundice, Joint pain, Muscle pain, Myalgia, Myopathy, Nephrolithiasis, Neutropenia, Peripheral neuropathy, Pneumonia, PR interval prolongation, Oral ulcerations, Taste perversion, Upper respiratory tract infections. All listed under "Adverse Effects of Antiretroviral Drugs", available at:

lists the drugs responsible as inhibitors of: CYP3A, Integrase, Nucleoside Reverse Transcriptase (NRTIs), Non-Nucleoside Reverse Transcriptase (NNRTIs), and Protease (PIs). *HIV InSite* adds Chemokine Coreceptor Antagonists, Fusion Inhibitors and Pharmocokinetic Enhancers.[24]

There are immediate problems with my presentation of this data. Not all of these drugs will give all of these symptoms to all of their consumers all of the time. Also, don't all medications have a long list of horrific side effects that are really just there to stop drug companies being sued? So, if you die after taking their product, they can say: 'We publicised the risk'.

That's true. But here's a question, how many people do you know who have to be encouraged to take their heart medication? How many diabetics do you know that are so adversely affected by insulin that they have to take 'drug holidays' just so their body will recover or so they can make it to an important family event without collapsing? Welcome to the strange world of anti-HIV drugs.

The problem of patient adherence to any anti-HIV drug regime is acknowledged by the U.S. Department of Health and Human services as huge:

> After receiving an HIV diagnosis, about 75% of individuals are linked to care within 30 days. However,

---

http://hivinsite.ucsf.edu/InSite?page=ar-05-01 posted on October, 2012 by Ian McNicholl, PharmD, BCPS, accessed 6th October 2017. Edited as in note above.

[24] Alphabetic order is mine.

only 57% of persons who receive an HIV diagnosis are retained in HIV care. It is estimated that only approximately 55% of persons with diagnosed HIV are virally suppressed because of poor linkage to care and retention in care. The data for adolescents and young adults are even more sobering: only 51% of youth living with HIV receive a diagnosis, 68% are linked to care within 1 month, and 55% are retained in care. (AIDSinfo, October 2017)[25]

Once-daily regimens, including those with low pill burden (even if not one pill once daily), without a food requirement, and few side effects or toxicities, are associated with higher levels of adherence. (*ibid*)

I cannot find comparable data for patient adherence to an oral chemotherapy regime on the same website, however the *Journal of Oncology Practice* published in the same year a study entitled "Treatment Satisfaction and Adherence to Oral Chemotherapy in Patients With Cancer" which shows far higher adherence:

As measured by the Medication Event Monitoring System, patients took, on average, 89.3% of their prescribed oral chemotherapy over the 12 weeks. One quarter of the sample was less than 90% adherent, and women were more adherent than men (Jacobs *et al.*)[26]

---

[25] "Adherence to the Continuum of Care", under "Limitations to Treatment Safety and Efficacy", under "Guidelines for the Use of Antiretroviral Agents in Adults and Adolescents Living with HIV", available at: https://aidsinfo.nih.gov/guidelines/html/1/adult-and-adolescent-arv/30/adherence – posted October 2017, accessed October 2017.

[26] Jaimie M. Jacobs, Nicole A. Pensak, Nora J. Sporn, James J. MacDonald, Inga T. Lennes, Steven A. Safren. Ellipsis mine. Posted May 2017, accessed October 2017. Available at: http://ascopubs.org/doi/full/10.1200/JOP.2016.019729

If you are outraged that I am not comparing like with like, you are quite justified in this feeling. People diagnosed with HIV are expected to put up with these officially acknowledged side effects from anti-HIV drug treatment regimes for the rest of their lives. In stark contrast is the humane advice from Cancer Research UK:

> A course of chemotherapy usually takes between 3 to 6 months. [...] During a course of treatment, you usually have between 4 to 8 cycles [...] After each round of treatment you have a break, to allow your body to recover. So if your cycle last 4 weeks, you may have treatment on the 1st, 2nd and 3rd days and then have nothing from the 4th to the 28th day.[27]

It must be said that some HIV researchers are beginning to admit the dangers of continual dosage of such highly toxic drugs and to advocate at least further study into structured treatment interventions, also known as 'drug holidays'. Published this year (2017) "The Continuous Controversy of Treatment Interruption" by Douglas Ward, MD (supported by "an unrestricted educational grant from: BMSVirology™ Bristol-Myers-Squibb Company, Boehringer Ingelheim, GlaxoSmithKline", all anti-HIV drug manufacturers) concludes:

> Even as patients' options for safe and effective treatment expand, the rule of maximally suppressive antiretroviral

---

[27] "Your Chemotherapy Plan", available at: www.cancerresearchuk.org/about-cancer/cancer-in-general/treatment/chemotherapy/planning/your-chemotherapy-plan?_ga=2.206117843.1919219939.1508850858-55721121.1508850858 – posted 2015, accessed October 2017. Ellipsis mine.

therapy for life is being vigorously reexamined from many quarters. If the same, or better, outcomes are possible with fewer drugs, or reduced total exposure to drugs, there can be little argument that less is more. Overall, the findings reviewed above indicate that partial or total interruption of therapy may be of real benefit to some patients in some situations. With hope, ongoing research will remove significant existing uncertainties as scientists zero in on the precise combinations of clinical, immunologic, virologic, and pharmacologic circumstances under which such approaches are unambiguously useful. Only then will we be able to employ them with confidence for the greater benefit of our patients.[28]

It is, of course, only to be expected that a biomedical researcher of Dr Ward's standing counsels caution in the interpretation of pharmaceutical findings. However, given the known life-threatening side effects of 'maximally suppressive antiretroviral therapy for life', one is left to wonder whether waiting for identification of 'precise combinations' of circumstances – to ensure that 'fewer drugs, or reduced total exposure' are 'unambiguously useful' when 'there can be little argument that less is more' – is really in the interest of those suffering from this iatrogenic harm.

---

[28] www.medscape.org/viewarticle/450726 – posted October 2017, accessed October 2017. For transparency, I quote the conclusion in full. I have inserted the colon and commas in the sentence regarding pharmaceutical company funding whereas the website simply has a cycle of their three logos.

HIV AS HARMLESS; AIDS AS INCOHERENT

Mere mention of the name of the scientist who is most famous for the claims of this chapter heading is the litmus test of HIV/AIDS paradigm affiliation. The established view of the biomedical-pharmaceutical Inquisition is exemplified by this quote from a post entitled "Pity poor Peter Duesberg" on the blog *Respectful Insolence* whose author, Mr David Gorski, describes himself as "a humble surgeon/ scientist" and writes under the pseudonym Orac:

> Back in the 1980s, he was on the top of the world, scientifically speaking. A brilliant virologist with an impressive record of accomplishment, publication, and funding, he seemed to be on a short track to an eventual Nobel Prize. Then something happened. The AIDS epidemic happened. Something about the AIDS epidemic led this excellent scientist in the late 1980s to fall directly into pseudoscience and crankery by latching onto and promoting the idea that HIV does not cause AIDS.[29]

I must say that this description is rather generous for its genre. Dr Kendrick refers to far more insidious attacks:

> Now, you can disagree with Duesberg if you like, and many people do. You can marshal your scientific arguments and engage him in debate. Or you can do what is generally done to those who hold ideas that do not fit with that of the authorities. You attack. In this case you call him a homophobic, racist, narcissistic,

---

[29] http://scienceblogs.com/insolence/2009/09/15/pity-poor-peter-duesberg-even-medical-hy/ – posted 2009, accessed October 2017.

nazi-sympathising, mass-murderer – one who also casually insults the disabled.

That, I think, is the royal flush of insults. (Kendrick/2014/125)[30]

The critique of Professor Duesberg by Seth Kalichmann, Professor of Psychology at the University of Connecticut, in his *New Humanist* article, "How to spot an AIDS denialist", is mild by comparison:

> In rare examples, denialist experts have a history of credible science only to have later gone off the deep end. The most credentialled AIDS denialists are Nobel Laureate Kari [*sic*] Mullis, who developed the PCR technology for sequencing the genetic code, and Peter Duesberg, Professor of Biochemistry and Molecular Biology at the University of California-Berkeley and member of the National Academy of Science. Although credentialled, neither is credible.[31]

"Crazy old Duesberg" is the view of some graduate students on campus reported by Garry Abrams of the *Los Angeles Times*, whose article, "Hero or Heretic? : Peter Duesberg, One of the Country's Top Virus Specialists, Risks Reputation With Theory That HIV Doesn't Cause AIDS", starts with this description:

---

[30] Kendrick/2014/124: "An on-line article by Jeanne Bergman for AIDStruth.org is the best concentrated example of character assassination that I have ever come across. In this passage she has adapted a *Newsweek* article entitled "*Newsweek* exposes Duesberg's psychopathology", which was written by Interlandi".

[31] https://newhumanist.org.uk/articles/2165/how-to-spot-an-aids-denialist – posted 2009, accessed October 2017. Gloss mine.

> BERKELEY – Peter Duesberg is learned, charming and urbane. He is a member of the National Academy of Sciences, an august body that does not elect underachievers. […]
>
> But for many of his peers, microbiologist Duesberg is the devil in disguise.[32]

Not for all. Professor Sir Andrew McMichael, learned, patrician and urbane, in a talk given to Glasgow Skeptics entitled, "Does HIV cause AIDS?", dismisses him as "a chemist".[33] Then bases almost the entirety of his presentation on refuting Professor Duesberg's claims. So, though some consider him, using Lady Caroline Lamb's famous judgement on Lord Byron, "mad, bad and dangerous to know", and others at best a "maverick" (Kalichman, *op. cit.*) for anyone who wants to understand contemporary objections to the HIV causes AIDS paradigm it is necessary to be clear about what Professor Duesberg continues to contend. It is also necessary to be clear about why he continues to contend it. His core contention is the following:

> HIV-positives actually have no reason to fear. As with uninfected people, those who stay off recreational drugs and avoid AZT will never die of "AIDS." Antibody-positive people can live absolutely normal lives.

---

[32] http://articles.latimes.com/1991-05-21/news/vw-2451_1_peter-duesberg – posted 1991, accessed October 2017, ellipsis mine.

[33] https://www.youtube.com/watch?v=VOeE8YsSZM4 – posted 2012, accessed October 2017. Dr Gallo (whom Professor McAndrew quite probably has read) says the same thing but has the grace to qualify this statement: "Duesberg is a chemist, a molecular virologist" (Gallo/1991/291).

> Worldwide, seventeen million of the eighteen million HIV-positives certainly do. Those at real risk of AIDS could help their fate if they were only informed that recreational drugs cause AIDS. And those with AIDS could recover if they were informed that AZT and its analogs inevitably terminate DNA synthesis, and thus life. (Duesberg & Ellison/1996/462)

The above quotation is from *Inventing the Aids Virus*, a closely-argued 722-page tome filled with detailed references and appendices, by Peter H. Duesberg, Professor of Molecular and Cell Biology at the University of California, Berekely, and Bryan J. Ellison who was his research assistant and a doctoral student there.[34]

There are three usual objections to Professor Duesberg's contention: drug-free AIDS in Africa, drug-free AIDS in infected haemophiliacs and drug-free AIDS in gay men.

Haemophiliacs

The various positions on the second are easiest to summarise. Dr Gallo, writing in 1991, makes a prediction that should be verifiable:

> Hemophilacs also make up a small percentage of infected people, although now that the blood supply has

---

[34] "Mr. Ellison did not participate in the final editing of the book or the preparation of the appendices." (Duesberg & Ellison/1996/Copyright page). "Bryan Ellison, Duesberg's former research assistant and original co-author, became disenchanted with Duesberg's and his publisher's insistence on careful documentation and self-published his own version under the title *Why We Will Never Win the War on AIDS* in 1994." (Duesberg & Ellison/1996/Publisher's Preface vii-viii).

been protected, blood-transfusion cases of AIDS will gradually decline and should approach zero in most industrialized regions of the world. (Gallo/1991/229)

Professor Duesberg counters this prediction in his first footnoted sentence in *Inventing the Aids Virus*:

> Even the screening of the nation's blood supply has not led to any notable reduction in AIDS-defining diseases (including pneumonia, candidiasis, and lymphoma) nor in death rates among blood transfusion recipients, including hemophiliacs. (Duesberg & Ellison/1996/462)

The footnoted reference is to Professor Duesberg's own work, published in 1992.[35] Since blood screening was variously instituted by various countries since the mid-1980s,[36] this short period may not give a clear picture of the effect of HIV-infected blood on haemophiliacs. However, by 2010, it was officially accepted that HIV transmission by blood transfusion was almost non-existent in the USA:

> A report published in the October 22 edition of the Centers for Disease Control and Prevention's *Morbidity and Mortality Weekly Report (MMWR)* describes the first known case of HIV transmission from a blood transfusion since 2002.

---

[35] "AIDS acquired by drug consumption and other noncontagious risk factors", *Pharmacology and Therapeutics*, 55 (1992): 201-277. Available at: www.ncbi.nlm.nih.gov/pubmed/1492119 – posted 1992, accessed October 2017.

[36] "Rare Case of Transfusion-Transmitted HIV Infection Reported", available at: www.hemophilia.org/Newsroom/Blood-Safety-News/Rare-Case-of-Transfusion-Transmitted-HIV-Infection-Reported – posted 2010, accessed October 2017.

> Enhanced screening, including the use of thorough questionnaires to exclude possible HIV-exposed donors and highly sensitive lab tests to identify infected blood donations, have reduced the risk of blood-borne HIV transmission dramatically. The report stated that [...] the risk for acquiring HIV infection through blood transfusion today is estimated conservatively to be one case in 1.5 million procedures.[37]

So, for Dr Gallo's 1991 prediction to come true, there should be a knock-on effect in the number of cases of AIDS. A number of factors complicate this easy prediction, as the conclusion of a 21-year Canadian study shows:

> The death rate among HIV-infected individuals with hemophilia in Canada reached a peak in 1993 and then subsequently declined following the introduction of effective antiretroviral therapy. The death rate began to plateau as of 1999, albeit at a rate higher than in the pre-HIV era. This excess mortality was due largely to the relative increase in the number of non-AIDS-related deaths, in particular, deaths due to liver disease.
>
> Recent data from other national hemophilia registries have shown a similar increase in the proportion of deaths due to liver disease and other non-AIDS-related deaths. Our cohort, with more than 21 years of follow-up, lends support to the importance of liver disease as an ongoing

---

[37] *Ibid*, italics original, ellipsis mine.

[38] "Mortality rates and causes of death among all HIV-positive individuals with hemophilia in Canada over 21 years of follow-up" by Donald M. Arnold, Jim A. Julian and Irwin R. Walker for the Association of Hemophilia Clinic Directors of Canada. Available at: www.bloodjournal.org/content/108/2/460?sso-checked=true – posted 2005, accessed October 2017.

cause of morbidity and mortality in this cohort of HIV and HCV co-infected individuals with hemophilia. With the introduction of HAART in Canada between 1995 and 1997, overall mortality and deaths due to AIDS has decreased, while deaths due to liver disease have increased. Liver disease may soon dominate as the most important cause of death among HIV-positive patients with hemophilia.[38]

In the UK, The Haemophilia Society has an on-going campaign involving the UK Government enquiry into "contaminated blood and blood products", as a report by Jefferson Courtney on their website explains. A key issue is the perceived partiality of the UK Department of Health in leading this enquiry, which the CEO is reported to have questioned on behalf of the Society. The same report has a summary of the contamination in the UK:

> In the 1970s and 1980s around 5,000 people with haemophilia and other bleeding disorders were multiply-infected with HIV, Hepatitis B and C and a range of other blood-borne viruses. Over 2,400 people have since died and of the 1,200 people infected with HIV less than 250 are still alive. [...]

> In the 1970s treatment of haemophilia and other bleeding disorders with fresh-frozen plasma and cryoprecipitate that contained the missing proteins was replaced with a new product, factor concentrate [...] such as factor 8 [...]

> Blood and blood products were known to transfer viruses such as Hepatitis [...] they were pooled using the new techniques. [...] products were increasingly imported from the United States. In the US, high-risk paid donors were used as well as being collected in prisons

> increasing the risk of contamination with blood-borne viruses.
>
> These risks were ignored by leading clinicians and Government [...] Pharmaceutical companies and leading clinicians did not appropriately share, or even hid, information about risks from patients and patient groups. Thousands of people were infected with deadly viruses during this time.[39]

This report does not let Professor Duesberg and fellow dissidents/ denialists off the hook in explaining apparently fatal HIV transmission by blood. However it does make clear that a reputable patient welfare society considers governments and pharmaceutical companies capable of cover-ups in their own financial and political interests rather than admitting the unjustifiable risks they have taken.

Professor Duesberg, while heartily concurring with this opinion of the conflict between the interests of patients and those of governments and pharmaceutical companies, explains this apparently fatal HIV transmission by blood differently, that blood transfusion is itself immunosuppressive, using seven presenting characteristics:

> 1) The increased life span of American hemophiliacs in the two decades before 1987, although 75% became infected by HIV – because factor VIII treatment, begun in the 1960s, extended their lives and simultaneously

---

[39] ""Clear Conflict of Interest" in DH Involvement in Contaminated Blood Inquiry", available at: http://haemophilia.org.uk/2017/10/09/clear-conflict-interest-dh-involvement-contaminated-blood-inquiry – posted October 2017, accessed October 2017. Ellipsis mine.

disseminated harmless HIV. After 1987 the life span of hemophiliacs appears to have decreased again, probably because of widespread treatment with the cytotoxic anti-HIV drug AZT.

2) The distinctly low, 1.3-2%, annual AIDS risk of hemophiliacs, compared to the higher 5-6% annual risk of intravenous drug users and male homosexual aphrodisiac drug users – because transfusion of foreign proteins is less immunosuppressive than recreational drug use.

3) The age bias of hemophilia-AIDS, i.e. that the annual AIDS risk increased 2-fold for each 10-year increase in age – because immunosuppression is a function of the lifetime dose of foreign proteins received from transfusions.

4) The restriction of hemophilia-AIDS to immunodeficiency diseases – because foreign proteins cannot cause non-immunodeficiency AIDS diseases, like Kaposi's sarcoma.

5) The absence of AIDS diseases above their normal background in sexual partners of hemophiliacs – because transfusion-mediated immunotoxicity is not contagious.

6) The occurrence of immunodeficiency in HIV-free hemophiliacs – because foreign proteins, not HIV, suppress their immune system.

7) Stabilization, even regeneration, of immunity of HIV-positive hemophiliacs by long-term treatment with pure factor VIII. (Duesberg/1994/49, paragraphing mine)

Conversely, Dr Gallo, writing three years earlier, to disprove a fungal co-factor of AIDS, claims that factor VIII was the problem, citing "James Curran of the Centres for Disease Control":

> More decisively, we knew from Curran and others that some hemophiliacs got AIDS from infusions consisting solely of Factor VIII, the clotting factor absent from their own blood. This blood-derived factor is filtered in a manner that would exclude fungi but it would not exclude a virus. (Gallo/1991/188)[40]

Dr Gallo provides no references for this (or any other) claim in this book but Professor Duesberg notes that Dr Montagnier proposed a mycoplasma (fungal-like bacterium) as a co-factor of AIDS after Professor Duesberg published in 1989 his first instalment of a planned debate between himself and the famous French HIV researcher in *Research in Immunology*, a debate which Dr Montagnier never joined (See: Duesberg & Ellison/1996/241-243).

In their highly technical (1994) paper, "Factor VIII, HIV and AIDS in haemophiliacs: an analysis of their relationship", the Perth Group present detailed empirical evidence to support their contention that neither the presence of virus-like particles, positive hybridization signals for 'viral' RNA, RT or p24 can be considered specific to HIV (Papadopulos-Eleopulos *et al.*/1994/30-34) and conclude (the section on viral isolation):

> This is as close a proof as one can get that what has been called HIV infection in haemophiliacs is not caused by an exogenous [of outside origin] retrovirus to which haemophiliacs have been exposed by the administration

---

[40] Dr Gallo *may* be referring to "Curran, J.W., D.N. Lawrence & H. Jaffe, 1984. Acquired immunodeficiency syndrome (AIDS) associated with transfusions, N. Engl. J. Med. 310: 69-75." – the first reference listed in Harris/1996.

of factor VIII preparations. (Papadopulos-Eleopulos *et al.*/1994/34, gloss mine)

Africans

Professor Stewart (1994/170) notes that the official conceptualisation of AIDS is unstable:

> the original empirical classification by the US/CDC accepted internationally in 1983 was expanded in 1987 to schedule and range of neoplasms, infections, malnutrition and dementia in which seropositivity to HIV, with or without risk-group identification, or these symptoms without seropositivity in risk groups were made eligible for classification as AIDS. This increased the size of the epidemic in the USA by about 27%.

1987 was also the year in which the toxic anti-HIV drug AZT was licensed, making estimations of cause and effect very complex, as the subsequent steep rise in cases of AIDS (rather than HIV) was certainly caused by the new classification but may also mask the fatal effect of the drug. There was another reclassification:

> To this list of 'indicator' diseases, a further revision in 1992, synchronous with identical changes in the International Classification of Diseases, added cancer of the cervix, tuberculosis and other diseases in persons who are seropositive. This has already added numerous females to the incidence of AIDS (*ibid*)

In the UK, we call this 'moving the goalposts'. It surely must become quite difficult to attempt to cure a disease when it is actually a collection of diseases loosely grouped together in a syndrome and the demarcation of that grouping keeps changing.

Steven B. Harris, M.D. – who deserves respect for being "the only medical scientist who agreed to defend the hypothesis that HIV is sufficient to cause AIDS" (Duesberg/1996/2) in a book written against that hypothesis – also takes issue with the definition of AIDS:

> epidemiological criteria implicate HIV as the casual agent in all AIDS cases, so long as AIDS is defined very narrowly (and most usefully) as the newly epidemic syndrome of life-threatening immune *failure* (*not* mild immune suppression) which occurs in certain groups of body-fluid exposed people at risk for an acquired infectious disorder. (Harris/1996/234, emphasis original)

Professor Duesberg's explanation of 'AIDS-related' disease in Africa does not keep to this narrow definition, as he sees it as neither new, epidemic, nor limited to certain demographic groups. Dr Duh accounts for the disparity in apparent mode of spread of HIV in Africa and Europe/ North America by his rather naive view of the prevalence of homosexuality (and perhaps of IV drug use):

> The two leading risk behaviors for AIDS – homosexual activity and IV drug use – in the Americas and Europe are rare (if not absent) in most African countries. (Duh/1991/55)

Whatever the etiology or extent of immune suppression or failure, Dr Duh also finds reports of African mortality from AIDS exaggerated:

> Even if one assumes that AIDS is grossly underreported – say only 10% of cases are reported – the death rate from AIDS is still relatively small. (Duh/1991/54)[41]

But can it really be claimed that 'AIDS is grossly underreported' in Africa? It seems that the reverse is true. Firstly, because the symptomology of AIDS in Africa is so similar to that of other prevalent conditions:

> Studies in several Central African countries indicate a relationship between endemic conditions and AIDS symptoms in children. The most common associations are malnutrition and anemia. Malnourished and anemic children tend to have pneumonias, diarrhea, oral candidiasis, lymphadenopathy, and dermatitis more frequently. (Duh/1991/60)

Secondly, because these conditions which Dr Duh sees as cofactors of AIDS are also among its defining diseases. Even in the case of a patient who has a negative result to an HIV test. Dr Duh (1991/67) makes this point explicitly: "there could be overreporting in some situations when the Bagui criteria (WHO, 1986) are used to identify AIDS cases."

Dr Duh goes on to explain the difficulty in distinguishing the symptoms of AIDS from those of other, endemic, diseases:

> For example, severe weight loss could be due to lack of adequate nutrient intake (or other respiratory infections);

---

[41] Duh (*ibid*) backs up this statement with data from a 1987 medical article, "Group-specific component and HIV infection. *Lancet*, p.1287", by Dr Konotey-Ahulu of Cromwell Hospital, London.

persistent cough could be due to tuberculosis in the absence of HIV infection; and chronic diarrhea is not uncommon in many African countries. (Duh/1991/67)

The World Health Organisation later admitted that, "the original WHO clinical case definitions for AIDS in children are not very sensitive or specific."[42] Dr Duh points out the risk of misdiagnosis:

> Studies in Zaire have shown that only 59% of AIDS cases diagnosed by the Bagui criteria had HIV infection. Tuberculosis was the most common illness by which false positive diagnoses of AIDS were made [...]; TB gives many of the same signs as used in the Bagui clinical definition of AIDS. (Duh/1991/67, ellipsis mine)

These criteria have since been updated but the WHO still lists TB as the most common killer:

> Tuberculosis (TB) killed 390 000 people living with HIV in 2015. It is the number one cause of death among people with HIV in Africa, and a leading cause of death in this population worldwide. (WHO, 2016)[43]

In 1993, in Northern Tanzania, British investigative journalist Neville Hodgkinson interviewed Philippe and Evelyne Krynen who, childless in mid-life, had "trained in France as nurses,

---

[42] "Who Case Definitions of HIV for Surveillance and Revised Clinical Staging and Immunological Classification of HIV-Related Disease in Adults and Children", available at: www.who.int/hiv/pub/guidelines/HIVstaging150307.pdf – posted 2007, accessed 11th October 2017.

[43] Under "HIV/AIDS", available at: www.who.int/features/qa/71/en/ – posted 2007, accessed 11th October 2017.

with a specialist qualification in tropical medicine, in order to dedicate the rest of their lives helping Third World orphans" (Hodgkinson/1996/352). In 1989 they had written a report for French charity *Partage Tanzanie*:

> *Voyage des Krynen en Tanzanie*, which was to prove a catalyst for world interest in the social impact of AIDS in Africa. It presented a dramatic picture: children alone in houses emptied of adults, or abandoned into the care of grandparents; a football team destroyed by the disease; old people sitting alone with their dead; black crosses painted at the entrances of AIDS-stricken homes.
>
> [...] it was a message that Western medical and charitable agencies, urgently wanting to alert people to the perceived dangers of HIV and AIDS, were more than ready to hear. (*ibid*, ellipsis & italics mine)

As the Krynens spent more time in the region of Kagera, "where Africa's first cases of AIDS were diagnosed" (*ibid*), "a very different picture of what was going on started to emerge compared with their first impressions" (Hodgkinson/1996/353):

> When appropriate treatment was given to villagers who became ill with complaints such as pneumonia and fungal infections that might have contributed to an AIDS diagnosis, they usually recovered.
>
> 'All of a sudden you have to put all you have been told about the disease in the garbage can, and try to reconsider', Evelyne said. 'The 15 villages we have looked at are in the most affected area of a region that is supposed to be at the epicentre of AIDS in Africa. When you listen to these people, you find they had been shocked by some deaths where the effects on the body

were very visual, with fungal infections and skin rashes. But these can be secondary effects of antibiotics, and the people who died with these conditions had all been treated before for conditions such as bronchitis. Nothing is sure, everything is just wind.' (*ibid*)

Hodgkinson summarises Philippe's explanation of the first reported AIDS deaths:

Most of the first deaths reported as AIDS were in young men trading in black-market goods in the aftermath of the Ugandan war. It started at the border, where people were dealing in drugs (*ibid*)

The Krynens learned that the 'orphans' were, in fact, children who did have parents but fostered by kin:

If Kagera is not, after all, in the grip of an epidemic of 'HIV disease', and if there is no AIDS, where have all the thousands of orphans come from? The answer, say the Krynens, is that most of the children are not orphans at all. Their final disillusionment was to discover that although many children are raised by their grandparents, that is a long-standing cultural feature of the region.

'The parents expatriate themselves a lot', Philippe explains. 'They move away from the region, sending a little money, returning little or never, but still have many children in the village. They are outwardly orphans, but raised by the grandmother or grandfather. It has always been like this; they may need help, but it has nothing to do with AIDS. Polygamy is also rampant here and they don't raise all the children they select very few and the others are just made and abandoned.' (Hodgkinson/1996/354)

Even the empty houses had an explanation:

'The houses that were empty were closed because they were the second or third homes of someone in Dar es Salaam', said Philippe. And the black crosses painted outside homes were leftovers from a population census, not a warning of AIDS. 'I learned this later. I have never seen a village with no adults, where children are like wolves in the forest. You know who is responsible for these stories? Party, *Partage*. We said that if we did not do something quickly, these villages would be emptied of adults and children would be like wild animals. The stories have been printed and reprinted, without the 'if'.' (Hodgkinson/1996/355, italics mine)

'My medical studies led me to believe that AIDS was devastating and the people who showed me the situation here reinforced this belief. I jumped into this, and made others believe it. And now I know that it was not true.' (Philippe Kyrnen, cited in Hodgkinson/1996/355)

Gay Men

Of the three usual objections to Professor Duesberg's contention that HIV is a harmless passenger virus and AIDS an incoherent set of unrelated diseases, the third (drug-free AIDS in gay men) is perhaps the most famous. Dr Gallo names Professor Duesberg explicitly in putting forward this objection:

> Duesberg has trouble with the concentration of AIDS in young gay men (in the United States and Europe), but HIV does concentrate in this group. He says viruses don't select by sex, but he is wrong: some do, and for many obvious and logical reasons. In fact, HIV is not the only virus more prevalent in this group. So are hepatitis B virus and some other sexually transmitted microbes. If enough members of a group are in more intimate

physical contact than others then, of course, there will be more infections in the group, particularly if the virus has much greater ease in its transmission by way of blood (more blood penetration is likely to take place in rectal sex than in vaginal sex). (Gallo/1991/291)

Dr Gallo also surmises that different ease of transmission by blood may account for the puzzling "extreme regionalisation of human retrovirus transmission" (Gallo/1991/229) and compares Thailand, where "HIV-1 is already spreading", to China, where "it is not a significant problem" (both, *ibid*) and states that:

Rio de Janeiro may have had one of the highest incidences of HIV in its blood supply early in the epidemic, as indicated by a small survey we carried out early in 1984, but many regions of South American were essentially HIV-free. We also tested blood from a number of Haitians shortly after we developed the blood test, and the HIV-positives were among the highest we had seen in blood from the early 1980s. But there are other Caribbean islands (for example Trinidad) where the rate was then much lower. I think this would be best explained by the better medical care and equipment available in Trinidad compared to Haiti, of the kind that ensures less likely contamination through blood (for example availability of sterile needles and syringes).

Other factors may also contribute to the discrepancy, such as ritualistic voodoo practices. (Gallo/1991/229-230)

Leaving aside the question of Dr Gallo's creative speculations on Voodoo, we turn now to Professor Duesberg's statistical study of drug-taking among gay men. This is a subject that makes many heterosexual people uncomfortable, even if they are allies of what used to be termed 'gay liberation'. It's one thing to publically lament the sickness and death of innocent babies or betrayed wives and girlfriends, as was very common in early AIDS reporting, but the moralistic corollary in the gutter press and from pious pulpits was always clear: gay men are hedonistic and their unnatural orgies have resulted in sickness and death. One way to counter this judgmental message was to state clearly: "All people with AIDS are innocent" as a 3x30 foot banner – hung over a Manhattan cultural centre by the New York AIDS activist art collective, Gran Fury – did in 1989.[44]

So for Professor Duesberg to seemingly blame AIDS on drugs, rather than disease, gave the impression that he was unsympathetic to a section of society already under fire for spreading 'the gay plague' to heterosexuals.[45] However, the question of whether or not Professor Duesberg or Dr Gallo, or any other researchers, have any particular sympathy for gay men (or Black people or haemophiliacs) is not as important as whether their scientific findings are helping in the fight against sickness and death.

---

[44] http://creativetime.org/projects/all-people-with-aids-are-innocent – posted November 2017, accessed November 2017.

[45] Colin Clews reports: "*The Australian* was one of the first newspapers to use the term (*"Gay plague" epidemic sweeping US'*, 17th July 1982)"
www.gayinthe80s.com/2014/04/1980s-hivaids-why-was-aids-called-the-gay-plague – posted April 2014, accessed November 2017.

Professor Duesberg's findings on drugs and AIDS are complex. He is an erudite and elite scientist and I cannot possibly summarise the 722 pages of his carefully written and referenced most famous work, *Inventing the AIDS Virus*, in a couple of paraphrased paragraphs when the original deserves to be read so that the context and nuance of his case against the CDC and the pharmaceutical industry is understood. Therefore, I have decided to focus on the link he identifies between the recreational use of (alkyl) nitrate 'poppers' and the prevalence of Kaposi's sarcoma in gay men:

> During the 1960s, male homosexuals discovered the aphrodisiac effects of nitrates. Receptive anal intercourse became less painful because the anal sphincter (muscle) would relax; therefore receptive men used far more of the drug than did their insertive partners. Nitrates also helped maintain erections and intensified orgasm, and some users even claimed a euphoric "high." (Duesberg & Ellison/1996/270)

As I started frequenting gay discos (as they were still known then) in the 1980s, I can testify to the ubiquitous cloud of poppers, usually amyl nitrate, in the air. Everyone knew of their physiological effect, the cult of the large penis and the general promiscuity meant that many gay men, especially those who were the passive sex partners of the well-endowed, used them frequently and even those of us who did not take them ourselves would be breathing them in on the disco floor or even (as happened to me on one occasion with an over-amorous suitor) having them shoved suddenly under our nose like Victorian smelling-salts. But such nitrates are not innocuous:

> By 1986 a statistical "AIDS link" to nitrate inhalants had become so convincing to public health officials that the sale of nitrates was banned by the United States Congress in 1988 (Public Health Law 100-690) and by the "Crime Control Act of 1990." However there are no reports that nitrate bans are ever enforced or that nitrate warnings are taken seriously. (Duesberg & Ellison/1996/271)

Considered not to fit the categorisation of psychoactive substances, poppers are not banned in the UK.[46] Yet the link is clear:

> The reactivity of nitrates easily compares with such toxins as carbon monoxide, the gas that suffocates its victims when a car engine is allowed to run in a closed garage. [...] At the height of the "popper craze," for example, a number of overdose victims arrived in hospital emergency rooms with as much as two-thirds of their hemoglobin chemically destroyed. Or to look at nitrates from another angle, a single dose can saturate the person using it with up to ten million nitrate molecules per cell in the body, leaving plenty of opportunity for damage. (Duesberg & Ellison/1996/271-272, ellipsis mine)

The link that Professor Duesberg refers to is to the most iconic AIDS disease: Kaposi's sarcoma. Unlike the mild skin

---

[46] See: "Ministers decide not to ban 'poppers'", available at: www.bbc.co.uk/news/uk-politics-35879663 – posted March 2016, accessed November 2017.

discolouration rarely seen in the general population of Mediterranean older men (Gallo/1991/260-261), the infamous lesions caused by the aggressive form of this tumour which commonly appeared in gay men old and young in the early days of AIDS became the graphic symbol of the syndrome in such Hollywood tearjerkers as *Philadelphia*.

Professor Duesberg records the brief moment when the US Centres for Disease Control took this link seriously:

> Recognizing the universal popularity of nitrates among homosexual men in 1981, the CDC was forced to consider this drug as one possible explanation of the emerging AIDS epidemic. [...] It did not even occur to them that nitrates could be toxic by themselves. Therefore they searched for a contaminated or bad batch of nitrates. [...] The CDC also assumed the effects would show immediately after using poppers, not after years of abuse, the way lung cancer and emphysema follow only after years of smoking tobacco. Naturally, no contaminated batch could ever be found, and the CDC dismissed the hypothesis altogether and thereafter focused its search entirely on infectious agents. (Duesberg & Ellison/1996/272, ellipsis mine)

In 1991 Dr Gallo describes this search as on-going:

I learned from epidemiologists that among HIV-infected people, homosexuals developed KS more than others. Later I heard that HIV-associated KS is on the decline relative to its rate a few years ago [...] Obviously, these findings suggested (but did not prove) that something in addition to HIV, even in the HIV-linked KS, was involved in the origin of KS. Could it be another accompanying microbe? Or was it some less specific co-factor(s)? (Gallo/1991/265, ellipsis mine)

By 1996, Professor Duesberg could state that the poppers-KS link was even clearer. Although, in the following extract from *Inventing the AIDS Virus*, Professor Duesberg notes 58 percent as a *decline* in reported use of poppers by gay men in San Francisco in 1984, this figure is still high enough to support any anecdotal evidence (including mine) that their use was frequent and widespread amongst gay men at the time of the announcement by the US Secretary of Health and Human Services (that HIV was the probable cause of AIDS) and had been for many years:

> Time has borne out the nitrate hypothesis of Kaposi's sarcoma. Early public health warnings about the drug's potential effects convinced many homosexual men to stop inhaling it. By 1984 only 58 percent of homosexual men in San Francisco said they used the drug on a regular basis, dropping to less than half that number by 1991. In parallel, the incidence of Kaposi's sarcoma also steadily dropped as a proportion of AIDS cases, from half of all AIDS reports in 1981 to only 10 percent by 1991. This has been the only AIDS disease to decrease this way, a change so shocking that the CDC itself briefly considered the possibility, in early 1991, that Kaposi's sarcoma might be a disease completely independent of AIDS and not caused by HIV. (Duesberg & Ellison/1996/273)

Poppers, at least in the UK, are not only not considered to be psychoactive substances by the government but also are not considered by their users (usually sexually passive or 'receptive' gay men) to be drugs – a word which in the UK, unless used by medical professionals, refers only to illegal psychoactive substances. Therefore, on completing a questionnaire regarding drug use, most gay men would not include amyl nitrate nor would they concur with being categorised as 'drug users'. The situation in the USA is different, where one buys 'drugs' from a 'drugstore'. Even so, there can be lack of clarity over who is actually consuming poppers (which in the USA are now illegal).

Professor Duesberg (1996/341-348) quotes a long letter, dated May 1995, from Raphael Sabato Lombardo, which illustrates this point. Discharged from the US Navy ten years previously after being diagnosed HIV positive, this young man (33 years old when writing) gives an extremely detailed and frank account of his sexual activity and of his total lack of illegal drug-taking. His point is a comparison of the length of his symptom-free survival time with that of "approximately 2 dozen" (*op. cit.*/341-344) friends similarly diagnosed who did take various illegal drugs, who suffered various symptoms and died sometime during the same period. Mr Lombardo mentions one woman (all the rest are gay men) who suffered on AZT, approved in 1987 (*op. cit.*/321-324), and died within 3 years (*op. cit.*/344-345). The website www.aidstruth.org, under the heading "Denialists who have died", comments on the death of Raphael Sabato Lombardo "a little over a year later" (June 1996):

> When asked about Lombardo's death, Duesberg wrote: "In hindsight, I think his letter was almost too good to be

true. I am afraid now, he described the man he wanted to be [e.g. that he did not use recreational drugs] and his Italian family expected him to be, but not the one he really was. I think he died from Kaposi's." (Source: Email to Richard Jeffreys from Peter Duesberg, Wednesday, April 05, 2006) (gloss original)

It is unclear whether (as many people diagnosed with HIV who end up in hospital, for whatever reason) he was persuaded in the end by medical staff and well-meaning family and friends, to succumb to AZT – eleven years after diagnosis which was a long survival time in those days. However, there is a simpler explanation, one that allows us to take this young man's honesty at face value. Although denying his own use of poppers, he lists in his sexual repertoire not only anal sex but fisting and that his friends had "heavy use" of poppers (Duesberg & Ellison/1996/345). Given the volatile nature of nitrate inhalants, as well as the risk of ingesting toxins by the ubiquitous use in gay discos of this drug during these years, the chances of the active sex partner inhaling some of the drug held under the nose of the passive sex partner are very high indeed. As the estimated average latency period for use of poppers to manifest as Kaposi's Sarcoma is "seven to ten years" (*op. cit.*/723), it is testament to Raphael Sabato Lombardo's otherwise healthy lifestyle that he managed to survive so long.

TESTING TESTING

> One day I pray that I will find the time to write or otherwise address the issue of the calamitous retreat from the habit of thinking in our country, the atrophy of meaningful intellectual engagement and communication, and the occupation of the realm of ideas largely by dearth of originality, superstition, opinionated prejudice, stereotypes and a herd mentality. (Pres. Thabo Mbeki)[47]

Henry Hermann Bauer, emeritus Professor of Chemistry and Science Studies at Virginia Polytechnic Institute and State University, defends the actions of the former South African president and questions the assumption that stavudine (a thymidine analogue DNA chain terminator, like AZT) can be described as 'life-saving'.

> The activist gurus of the Treatment Action Campaign (TAC) have long castigated President Mbeki and others for not providing the life-saving benefits of antiretroviral drugs to South Africans. But now the very same self-appointed experts, in collaboration with Médecins Sans Frontières (MSF) have asked the Gates Foundation not to support a clinical trial in which the relative benefits of tenofovir are to be compared with stavudine at 20 mg dosage – because stavudine is so toxic![48]

The letter Professor Bauer refers to is hardly reassuring about even the short-term effects of thymidine analogues such as AZT (no-

---

[47] President Thabo Mbeki in a letter to his biographer, Ronald Suresh Roberts, 1st January 2006. Available at: www.mbeki.org/profile-of-former-president-thabo-mbeki – posted 2016, accessed November 2017.

[48] https://hivskeptic.wordpress.com/2011/12/30/haart-is-toxic-mainstream-concedes-it-in-backhanded-ways – posted 2011, accessed November 2017.

one now seems to argue that their scattershot action which also wipes out opportunistic infections outweighs their toxicity in the long term) and is even more damning considering that it is written by people who do not question the hypothesis that HIV causes AIDS.[49]

ELISA & Western Blot

As we now know the deadly toxic nature of AZT, the main antiretroviral drug available at the time when Dr Duh was writing (and one he enthusiastically recommends) we may have more sympathy for those authorities – including President Thabo Mbeki of South Africa – who have raised concerns about the massive deployment of pharmaceutical drugs in Africa when there is such danger of misdiagnosis and false positive results from HIV tests:

> Serologic tests used in some African countries may contribute to a possible overestimation of AIDS/HIV infection. Many of the tests used earlier during the epidemic were inaccurate [...] Cross-reactivity of the HIV antigen with antigens of tropical organisms, such as the organism that causes malaria, continues to be a problem in some countries. Until such time that tests for HIV are purified, the potential for overestimating the problem will continue to exist. (Duh/1991/68-69, ellipsis mine)

---

[49] Letter available on *Médecins Sans Frontières* Access Campaign website at: www.msfaccess.org/sites/default/files/MSF_assets/HIV_AIDS/Docs/AIDS_Letter_MSFtoGatesStavudineTDFclinicaltrial_ENG_2011.pdf – posted 2011, accessed November 2017.

This problem has not gone away, as an explanation (that appears to me particularly convoluted) of the findings of a study done in 2011, on HIV test false positives in Kenya and Uganda, attempts to clarify:

> The phrase 'false positive paradox' describes our primary findings. When the incidence of any given condition is lower than a test's false positive rate, even tests that have a high specificity (i.e., low chance of giving a false positive in an individual case) will generate more false than true positives. [...] Therefore, as HIV prevention activities in at-risk populations are successfully implemented, true positive HIV results should decline, as the number of incident HIV infections decline, but false positives will occur as they are inherent to the testing assay itself and are not influenced by prevention efforts.[50]

I'm really not clear on why a test for HIV that yields a high rate of false positives, by a process apparently inherent to the assay itself, is considered reliable. I reproduce the entire Results paragraph from the Abstract of the same study:

> A total of 99,009 monthly HIV tests were performed; 98,743 (99.7%) were dual-rapid HIV negative. Of the 266 visits with ≥1 positive rapid result, 99 (37.2%) had confirmatory positive EIA results (true positives), 155 (58.3%) had negative EIA results (false positives), and

---

[50] "Frequency of False Positive Rapid HIV Serologic Tests in African Men and Women Receiving PrEP for HIV Prevention: Implications for Programmatic Roll-Out of Biomedical Interventions", available at:
www.ncbi.nlm.nih.gov/pmc/articles/PMC4401675 – posted April 2015, accessed October 2017. Ellipsis mine.

12 (4.5%) had discordant EIA results. In the active PrEP arms, over two-thirds of visits with positive rapid test results were false positive results (69.2%, 110 of 159), although false positive results occurred at <1% (110/65,945) of total visits.

If I understand these statistics correctly, 53% of test results indicating HIV antibodies (taken to mean the presence of HIV) were in fact false positives. So 155 people out of 266 were informed, erroneously, that they were 'HIV positive'. The fact that this number of people disappears in the larger figure – for all those who did the test whatever their result – seems to me irrelevant.[51] *Imagine if you were one of those 155 people.*

The EIA test is also known as ELISA; Dr Gallo explains the acronym:

> So, using the virus itself in the enzyme-linked immune absorbent assay (ELISA) test, Sarang could now conduct wide-spread serological testing of the general population for the presence of antibodies to the AIDS virus. Our first test group would include people from each of the three target groups: those with AIDS, those in high risk categories, and a control population.
>
> We quickly determined that even with a quality virus and a stable single type of cell-producing virus (therefore less variable background "noise"), the ELISA could

---

[51] I also note the following information (usually cited under 'possible conflict of interest'): "This work was supported by The Bill and Melinda Gates Foundation (grant OPP47674) and the National Institute of Mental Health of the US National Institutes of Health (grant R01 MH095507)." (*ibid*)

sometimes give false positive or false negative results. A confirmatory test was essential. (Gallo/1991/183)[52]

Dr Corbitt gives the same *caveat*, with slightly less convoluted statistics, about false positives in HIV testing:

> As the prevalence of infection in the population increases the incidence of false positives decreases. At a prevalence of 1.0 per cent the same EIA [ELISA] test will have a PPV [Positive Predictive Value] of 83.4 per cent and at a prevalence of 10 per cent the PPV will have risen to 98.2 per cent.
>
> Thus in test populations with a high prevalence of HIV infection a single test for antibody will detect a large proportion of true positives and yield relatively few false positives. Use of a single screening assay on a population with a low prevalence of HIV infection is simply not acceptable since many of the 'reactive' results obtained will be false positives. The way round this problem is to use additional EIAs or supplementary tests (Western Blot, LIA)[53] to retest reactive sera. (Corbitt/2001/30, gloss mine)

Paraphrasing Dr Corbitt, as prevalence of reported HIV *decreases*, he expects an associated *increase* in false positives from

---

[52] 'Sarang' is Dr M.G. Sarngadharan, then "Director of the Department of Cell Biology, Advanced Bioscience Laboratories, Inc., Kensington, Maryland." (Gallo/1991/caption on a photo between pp.148-149)

[53] LIA refers to line immunoassay, a development of ELISA, also known as 'lineblot'. Niel Constantine, PhD, University of Maryland School of Medicine, states: "The use of LIA is popular in Europe, but these tests have not been licensed for use in the United States. A number of reports have verified that the accuracy is equivalent to the Western blot." Available at:
http://hivinsite.ucsf.edu/InSite?page=kb-02-02-01#S6.4X – posted May 2006, accessed November 2017.

HIV antibody tests. His concern appears to be that an increasing number of members of the general population (i.e. persons outside the 'risk groups') will find themselves falsely diagnosed with HIV and put on antiretroviral drugs – whose toxicity is acknowledged. As for persons who happen to be Black, or gay men, or haemophiliacs, or IV drug users, or Haitians, the good doctor reassures us that there is a higher possibility that they will be positive anyway, so we don't need to worry about the growing number of those who are diagnosed in error.

The Western Blot test is considered so unreliable that it is no longer used in most post-industrialised countries. Biomedical researchers at McMaster University, Ontario, Dr Tahrin Mahmood (now at the University of Toronto) and Professor Ping-Chang Yang, explain the problems:

> Even though the procedure for western blot is simple, many problems can arise, leading to unexpected results. The problem can be grouped into five categories: (1) unusual or unexpected bands, (2) no bands, (3) faint bands or weak signal, (4) high background on the blot, and (5) patchy or uneven spots on the blot.[54]

Dr Gallo (1991/223) injects some rare humour into this bleak topic, explaining that the name of the technique continues a biomedical researcher in-joke:

---

[54] "Western Blot: Technique, Theory, and Trouble Shooting", available at: www.ncbi.nlm.nih.gov/pmc/articles/PMC3456489 – posted September 2012, accessed October 2017.

For several years, scientists had used a certain procedure called a Southern Blot when used for DNA (named after Ed Southern of Edinburgh) and a Northern Blot when used for RNA (named so for obvious reasons).

American investigative journalist Celia Farber summarises information from "Is a Positive Western Blot Proof of HIV Infection?", published in the biomedical journal *Bio/Technology* in 1993, which explains that these bands refer to proteins (and glycoproteins):

> The Western Blot detects patterns of proteins thought to be specific to HIV. These are specified as 'p' for protein, followed by a molecular weight. HIV is recognized by proteins p24, p17, gp41, gp120, etc. (Farber/1996/344)

The Abstract, of this *Bio/Technology* article, is here in full:

> It is currently accepted that a positive Western blot (WB) HIV antibody test is synonymous with HIV infection and the attendant risk of developing AIDS. In this communication we present a critical evaluation of the presently available data on HIV isolation and antibody testing. This evidence indicates that: (1) the antibody tests are not standardized; (2) the antibody tests are not reproducible; (3) the WB proteins (bands) which are considered to be encoded by the HIV genome and to be specific to HIV may not be encoded by the HIV genome and may in fact represent normal cellular proteins; (4) even if the proteins are specific to HIV, because no gold standard has been used to determine specificity, a positive WB may represent nothing more than cross-reactivity with non-HIV antibodies present in AIDS patients and those at risk. We conclude that the use of antibody tests as a diagnostic and epidemiological tool

for HIV infection needs to be reappraised. (Papadopulos-Eleopulos *et al.*/1993)

This article is co-authored by biophysicist Dr Eleni Papadopulos-Eleopulos, emergency physician Dr Valendar F. Turner and pathologist Dr John M. Papadimitiou, who – as they work at the Royal Perth Hospital, Western Australia – are often known as (the core of) 'the Perth Group'. Rather than simply question the possibility of the infectious nature of HIV, the Perth Group – whom Professor Duesberg (1996/252) describes as "the most outspoken medical team to challenge the HIV hypothesis" – question the proof for its very existence.

HIV AS INEXISTENT; AIDS AS INCOHERENT

Dr Kary B. Mullis, co-winner of the 1993 Nobel Prize in Chemistry, sought a reference for the verification of the hypothesis that HIV causes AIDS in the form of a now (in)famous statement:

> In 1988 I was working as a consultant at Specialty Labs in Santa Monica, setting up analytic routines for the Human Immunodeficiency Virus (HIV) […] when I found myself writing a report on our progress and goals for the project, sponsored by the National Institutes of Health, I recognized that I did not know the scientific reference to support a statement I had just written: "HIV is the probable cause of AIDS". (Mullis in Duesberg & Ellison/1996/xi, ellipsis mine)

Dr Mullis goes on to state that his search was in vain. The search for verification (or not) of this hypothesis has perhaps been most famously conducted by the Perth Group, who stated in 1997:

> Since there is no such data proving the origin of either "HIV" proteins or antibodies, and since there is ample evidence that reactions between "HIV" proteins and "HIV" antibodies are non-specific, including reactivity caused by organisms and agents to which AIDS patients and those at risk are subjected, it is vital for the scientific community to utilise valid methods in order to prove whether the "HIV" proteins and antibodies arise as the result of a new, unique, exogenously acquired retrovirus.[55]

---

[55] www.theperthgroup.com/SCIPAPERS/epcurmedres97.html – posted 1997, accessed October 2017.

We left 'Lucy' the retrovirus some chapters back. Perhaps by now, the various personal props that I used to illustrate this cartoon character version of HIV might be more familiar. If so, then we may be able to better understand the problems that the Perth Group have with the claims that 'Lucy' exists at all.

Without going into huge philosophical detail over the tricky relationship between ontology (the real nature of something) and epistemology (how we know about something's nature),[56] it now has to be admitted that no researcher really knows for certain what actually goes on in Mr Moody's office and still less about whether Lucy is at work there or not.

This is because researcher don't have a God's eye view. They can't simply take the roof off the building and peer in. All they can do is observe at a distance who or what goes into and out of the building (which we can imagine either as an organ or as an entire body) and hope, fondly, that the result either of their observation or of any intervention isn't structural collapse.

AZT is the SWAT team that storms the building and wipes out all life. Mission accomplished. Just in case Lucy, suspected terrorist, was about to abseil her clones (copies of viral RNA) out of the windows and start terrorising (infecting) another building.

---

[56] For those that do like that sort of thing, I recommend the bestselling metaphysical novels of the late Dr Robert M. Pirsig and my doctoral thesis (McManus/2011) which reflects on them.

Unfortunately, this also means that Mr Moody (DNA) is inhibited from carrying on with the business as usual of the office (cell).[57]

Mr Moody's office in this metaphor is a white blood cell (leucocyte or leukocyte in Greek) and, specifically, a lymphocyte. So, broadly, Mr Moody works in the Security section of the building (body). Some lymphocytes (B-cells) are stimulated by antigens (perceived security threats) to become plasma cells that produce specific antibodies (in the UK, we'd call these kind of Security staff 'bouncers'). However, Mr Moody's office is a CD4 T-cell, a 'helper', which means it coordinates 'killer' CD8 T-cells to neutralise the threat (antigens).[58]

As anti-HIV drugs are toxic, they are perceived as threats. So it's unsurprising that initially they cause T-cell counts to rise, before they too succumb to the toxins. Newer anti-HIV drugs are *less* lethal. At first. They deal with bodies suspected of harbouring HIV the way the Israeli army deals with homes suspected of harbouring terrorists. Nothing happens for a while, then BOOM! Building blown up (liver failure).[59] Another life in rubble. So how do these various killers aim

---

[57] "When it was studied, it was found that, unsurprisingly, AZT reduced the 'viral load' in AIDS. Frankly it would have been amazing if it had not, as all replication, of everything inside the human body, was being switched off." (Kendrick/2014/190).

[58] I apologise for this no doubt very inexact summary of the clear and very detailed information set out in my source: http://bme.virginia.edu/ley/leukocyctes.html – no date, accessed November 2017.

[59] See my footnote 38, above.

at the right target? Well, the problem is that we don't have any direct evidence of Lucy's existence or whereabouts. A smear of lipstick, a strand of hair (that may or may not be human) or a bit of leather that could as equally come off the couch as off Lucy's handbag.

Dr Mullis won his Nobel Prize "for his invention of the polymerase chain reaction (PCR) method",[60] which has been claimed (not by him) to prove the existence of HIV. Professor Duesberg explains the limitations of PCR when used in the hunt for HIV:

> The PCR is a technology that amplifies even the tiniest amounts of any specific DNA sequence, creating enough copies of the desired sequence for detection and analysis. This amounts to finding the proverbial needle of dormant HIV in a haystack of human DNA. But contrary to statements by some HIV scientists, this is not an isolation of the actual virus and does not fulfil Koch's second postulate. It is only the detection of dormant DNA genomes, or fractions of viral genomes, left behind from infections that occurred years earlier. (Duesberg & Ellison/1996/180)

Dr Mark Craddock (lecturing in Mathematics at the University of New South Wales at the time of his writing, then Senior Lecturer in the same subject at the University of Sydney) explains, in the Abstract of "Some mathematical considerations on HIV and AIDS", that in this use of PCR the numbers don't add up:

---

[60] www.nobelprize.org/nobel_prizes/chemistry/laureates/1993/mullis-facts.html – posted 1993, accessed October 2017.

Questions that have arisen about the virus include whether or not it is present in sufficient quantities to cause disease and whether or not AIDS is infectious. The former question has been applied to by new studies using the Polymerase Chain Reaction (PCR) technique that claim to detect very large quantities of virus in HIV+ patients at all stages of disease progression. I will examine these studies and show that they do not truly answer the criticisms that have been levelled. They in fact give rise to more questions than they answer. Predictions that one can make from them contradict the observed patterns of the disease. I will also argue that data based on the so called Quantitative Competitive PCR need to be treated with caution. (Craddock/2006/89)[61]

Dr Gallo (1991/278) takes up Professor Duesberg's point and summarises Koch's postulates (the following does not appear to be a direct quote and it is unclear if the parentheses and italics are Dr Gallo's or of the 18th century German medical researcher and pioneer of microbiology, Professor Robert Heinrich Hermann Koch):

1. The germ must be found in the *affected* tissue (the presumed site of the disease) in *all* cases of the disease. (At every site of disease tissue, we find the germ.)

---

[61] I have not 'shown the working' as, frankly, algebra and statistics at that level are beyond me and I simply would not know what to quote, after the plain English of the Abstract. For those who *do* understand them, see "Viral Load and the PCR: Why they can't be used to prove HIV infection", available at: http://helpforhiv.com/viralload.htm – published in *Continuum* November 2001, accessed November 2017 – which quotes and references Dr Craddock and other experts in these and related fields.

2. The germ must not occur in other diseases or as a fortuitous non-pathogenic agent. (In every case where we find the germ, we find the disease.)

3. It must be repeatedly isolated in pure form, free from other germs and from the host body. (We must be able to identify and study the germ on its own.)

4. The germ so isolated must be able to induce the disease anew and be re-isolated from the inoculated animal. (Every animal into which we introduce the germ must get the disease and yield new germs.)

Whether these famous postulates are still valid or not,[62] Dr Gallo agrees with Professor Duesberg that the hypothesis that HIV is the cause of AIDS violates them. Both Professor Duesberg and the Perth Group claim that the hypothesis that HIV is the cause of AIDS also violates some wise advice regarding scientific research that was given centuries before Koch's Postulates, by a mediaeval friar named William of Occam:

> Many scientists have adopted or reinvented Occam's Razor, as in Leibniz's "identity of observables" and Isaac Newton stated the rule: **"We are to admit no more causes of natural things than such as are both true and sufficient to explain their appearances."**
>
> The most useful statement of the principle for scientists is "when you have two competing theories that make

---

[62] Dr Gallo (1991/279) makes the point that these postulates are outdated, using TB as an example: "most infected persons are *healthy* carriers. Koch's postulates did not consider this notion, which is a central theme today in the study of almost all infectious diseases. In short, even for his classical work on TB, postulate number two was not fulfilled."

exactly the same predictions, the simpler one is the better."[63]

Straining the Imagination

The HIV hypothesis is certainly not simple. Investigating claims of 'family trees' of HIV strains as evidence of infection increasingly used in court to criminalise sex without a condom, when one partner has not disclosed a positive HIV antibody test result, I came across this headline on *Alphr*, an online popular science journal: "Scientists create 'three-in-one' antibody that attacks 99% of HIV strains". Abigail Beall, the author, has a *caveat*: "While this is a promising result, the treatment has only be [*sic*] tested on monkeys and the primate form of HIV".[64] In the same article, the author elucidates further:

> During trials, the anitbody [*sic*] protected monkeys from two forms of SHIV, the primate form of HIV, in 24 primates.
>
> It works by binding to three critical sites on the virus, making it harder for HIV to resist its attack. It is known as a 'broadly neutralising antibody' because it can attack many forms of HIV, even when the virus changes shape.

A distracted read of Ms Beall's breathless prose may miss the fact that 'the virus' referred to is *not* HIV and also that SHIV

---

[63] http://math.ucr.edu/home/baez/physics/General/occam.html – bold emphasis original; italics & paragraphing mine.

[64] Both: www.alphr.com/science/1007120/HIV-antibody – published online 22nd September 2017, accessed 7th December 2017.

(Simian/Human Immunodeficiency Virus) is a 'chimera' of SIV, officially harmless to humans and monkeys alike, and HIV, officially harmless to monkeys (and, unofficially, to humans). The 'official' conclusions (that 'SIV is not a monkey killer') I have quoted above, from the intrepid monkey researchers Wertheim and Worobey, corroborated by Professor Duesberg:

> Simian Immunodeficiency Virus (SIV), a monkey retrovirus, attracts most of the attention. But these animal diseases can be called "AIDS" only by stretching the definition to extremes. [...] the animal symptoms usually resemble the flu: The animals become sick within days or not at all, without long latent periods [...] In the wild, their cousins retain antibodies against SIV all their lives without ever becoming sick from the virus. (Duesberg & Ellison/1996/204, ellipsis mine)

Fascination with the strains of HIV is not limited to the breathless blogging of freelance popular science journalists. The Wikipedia user (author) who rejoices in the name 'Soupvector', and is revealed upon investigation to be one "Stuart Ray, M.D., a physician-scientist at Johns Hopkins University (JHU) School of Medicine", has a beautifully-sketched highly edited illustration of a few of the multitude of strains of HIV currently imagined to be in existence. It resembles the seedhead of a dandelion and, interestingly, has the strains of HIV-2 (mostly found in Africa) far apart from HIV-1 but very close to SIV. Indeed, he even has some strains of SIV branching off from those of HIV-2, indicating (no doubt) some kind of human-monkey interaction that any intrepid researcher in that field would find fascinating.[65]

I only became aware of the extent to which this charming illustration has been edited when I reviewed the published source of the data (the illustration itself is the creation of Soupvector): Los Alamos National Laboratory/ National Institutes of Health/ Dept. Of Health and Human Services. What I took to be genomic sequences of 63 diverse HIV strains span pages 160-223. Then I noticed the caption running alongside: "HIV Sequence Compendium 2016: HIV-2 Genomes". Then a note in the Introduction:

> Compared to HIV-1, fewer HIV-2 genomes have been sequenced, so we are able to include all available HIV-2 genomes, removing only problematic sequences and multiples from the same patient.[…]
>
> The HIV-2/SIVsmm family is presented together in spite of their different hosts, because their genomic structure is the same[66]

This is not terribly reassuring. If I understand this at all (and I don't claim to understand it at all well) the HIV-1 has even more strains than HIV-2, and SIV is basically identical to HIV-2! So, with the latest scare stories about 'recombinant' HIV rampaging through Cuba, among other locations,[67] the amount of diverse strains of HIV

---

[65] https://en.wikipedia.org/wiki/Subtypes_of_HIV – last online edit 4th December 2017, accessed 7th December 2017.

[66] www.hiv.lanl.gov/content/sequence/HIV/COMPENDIUM/2016/hiv2dna.pdf – no date (but clearly no earlier than 2016), accessed 7th December 2017. Ellipsis mine.

is high indeed! This means that the HIV-AIDS hypothesis has become even more unverifiable. Professor Duesberg explains why:

> The argument from speculation is used more often than any other [Ignoring the Facts; Inappropriate Models; Antibody Correlations]. It uses specialized terms that make it difficult for outsiders to understand, responding to any paradox with one untested assumption after another. For instance, if little of no HIV can be found in the body, scientists propose hidden reservoirs and special routes of infection. If only antibodies against HIV can be found, researchers call them "nonneutralizing" (or ineffective) antibodies and assert that the virus mutates too fast for the virus to keep up. If the virus does not make animals sick or kill cells in culture, then researchers claim that the virus somehow makes fine distinctions between humans and chimpanzees, something no other virus can do. All these hypotheses are constantly being disproved or shown to be irrelevant, but the reservoir of new evasions is inexhaustible. (Duesberg & Ellison/1996/205-206; gloss from titles on pp.199-208)

Prophetic words written in 1996. The HIV-AIDS hypothesis has only grown more complex. Dr Harris (1996/232) also notes this process in the philosophy of science:

> It has been observed by the late Karl Popper, noted philosopher of science, that [...] nearly any theory can be tinkered with after the fact, so that it continues to 'explain' all data.

---

[67] www.iflscience.com/health-and-medicine/highly-aggressive-new-strain-hiv-spreading-through-cuba/ – no date (but one source dated 2015), accessed 7th December 2017.

Strategies of Dissent

Although Professor Duesberg's claim, that HIV is harmless, and the Perth Group's contention, that HIV has never been proven to exist at all, may seem contradictory, I feel that they have a different focus. As someone who has neither medical or scientific qualifications nor the privilege of acquaintance with any of these erudite researchers, I can only give my general impression that the focus of Professor Duesberg's publications and public pronouncements in this field appears to be on the phenomena of AIDS, whereas that of the Perth Group appears to me to be on HIV.

This, unofficial and unsubstantiated personal view, may provide a possible explanation for Professor Duesberg's dismissal of condoms and 'safe sex'. Of course there are very good reasons, of both health and hygiene, as well as for prevention of pregnancy, for the use of condoms in both anal and vaginal sex (their use in oral sex is apparently a moot point) but Professor Duesberg's argument appears to be that if someone's immune system has already been gravely compromised by drugs (including anti-HIV drugs) then the use of a preventative measure for something that is not the cause of the present condition is not a priority.

Professor Duesberg is apparently also something of a joker and when the journal *Continuum* put up a reward for the isolation of HIV, he claimed it in an article, "Peter Duesberg Responds" published in the same journal in 1996. For technical reasons, he was not awarded the prize, as an editorial "Focus" section of the same issue explains:

> Because Prof. Duesberg's preferred technique for retroviral isolation does not fulfil the Pasteur Institute methodology (1973) which was the criterion of the *Continuum* isolation prize, it has not been possible to grant his claim to the prize, albeit he argues that other isolation techniques exist.[68]

That Professor Duesberg's motivation for this publication was not altogether jocular, but rather to rid the cause of distractions, he explains at the conclusion to his response to the response of the Perth Group (to his response to the competition!):

> the high standards of virus isolation from extracellular materials postulated by Papadopulos *et al.* and Hodgkinson may be relevant for crystallographers or chemists who want to analyze the structure of a virus, but are not relevant for functional isolation.
>
> In view of this I hope to liberate the minds of HIV dissidents from HIV for the cause that unites us all – the solution of AIDS. It seems tragic that over 99% of AIDS researchers study a virus that does not cause AIDS and that the few who don't are now engaged in a debate over the existence of a virus that doesn't cause AIDS.[69]

---

[68] "Global Concern on Viral Isolation" *Continuum* (July/August 1996) Vol. 4, No. 3 p.7. Available at: www.immunity.org.uk/wp-content/uploads/2013/06/v4n2.pdf – accessed November 2017.

[69] "Near Enough *is* Good Enough?" *Continuum* (February/March 1997) Vol.4, No. 5 p.26. Available at: www.immunity.org.uk/wp-content/uploads/2013/06/v4n5.pdf – accessed November 2017.

As far as I can follow this *extremely* erudite debate, at least one disagreement (I can't be certain it's the main one) is over the relative merits of functional and structural criteria for validation of viral isolation. Notwithstanding this frank exchange of views (which must be rather refreshing for all concerned as it is exactly this kind of debate that is lacking on HIV and AIDS) the beginning of Professor Duesberg's one page article shows his very gracious attitude towards his colleagues:

> I am honoured by the profound and passionate reactions of Hodgkinson, Lanka and Papadopulos-Eleopulos et al. to my letter on the existence or the non-existence of HIV

In the Summary of their own article, "Why *no* whole virus?" in the same issue (pp.27-30) the Perth Group respond with the same respectful tone (although with no less scientific rigour and with passion) emphasising that they are indeed on the same side:

> What does one have to do and how hard does one have to plead in order to obtain answers to fundamental questions regarding a retrovirus which has menaced the world and in whose name hundreds of thousands of people have died or been poisoned?
>
> For example:
>
> 1. How is it possible to transmit a cell-free retrovirus, "HIV", when it is accepted that:
>
> (i) gp 120 is absolutely necessary for the virus to enter the cell and for the "cycle of viral replication to begin";

(ii) to date nobody has reported the existence of cell-free particles with the dimensions of retroviral particles possessing knobs, that is, gp 120?

2. How can one claim that AIDS patients and those at risk are infected with a unique retrovirus, HIV, when to date nobody has even reported in fresh, cultured tissue, or tissue co-cultures, particles fulfilling the principal morphological and physical characteristics of retroviral particles?

We agree with Peter Duesberg that "the cause that unites us all" is finding a solution to AIDS. With this our aim we were among the first to put forward non-infectious factors as agents to explain AIDS in gay men and furthermore we were the first to propose a non-infectious theory with a unifying mechanism to explain the development of AIDS in all risk groups. Indeed, our theory also predicts a non-infectious explanation for the phenomena which others have inferred as "isolation" of a novel retrovirus from AIDS patients.

Before commenting on this debate, again, in 1999, the Perth Group explain the pragmatic reasons for their former strategy of letting the "facts to speak for themselves":

i. To facilitate publication;

ii. To avoid a split in the group [...] Also we could not exclude the possibility that the HIV theory of AIDS could be deconstructed without questioning the existence of HIV. ("The Last Debate", the Perth Group)[70]

---

[70] All www.theperthgroup.com/POPPAPERS/lastdebate.html – posted 1999, accessed November 2017, ellipsis mine.

In contrast to Professor Duesberg, the Perth Group appear to feel, perhaps rightly, that neither the general public nor the scientific community are listening to the drugs hypothesis as an alternative to HIV:

> If [...] we accept the existence of HIV, the debate could be endless, no matter how courageously one fights and what sacrifices one makes. In this regard Peter Duesberg's unprecedented contribution is a wise and timely reminder to all of us. (*ibid*, ellipsis mine)

Isolation of HIV

The Perth Group focus on taking issue with the claim that anyone, including Dr Gallo and Dr Montagnier, has ever isolated HIV.

> HIV is the main obstacle, indeed, the only obstacle, in deconstructing the HIV theory of AIDS. (*ibid*)

Under the subheading of Viral Isolation, a Perth Group paper, published by Professor Duesberg, refers to various HIV studies:

> In a paper published in the *Lancet* in 1984 entitled 'Isolation of a New Lymphotropic Retrovirus from two Siblings with Haemophila B, one with AIDS', Montagnier and his associates were the first to describe 'isolation of HIV' from haemophiliacs. (Papadopulos-Eleopulos *et al.*/1994/30)

The Perth Group paper adds other instances of 'isolation':

> Using similar methods, researchers from the CDC and the Children's Hospital of Los Angeles reported in 1985

> the isolation of HIV from 6 of 19 healthy seropositive [HIV antibody positive] haemophiliacs (Gomberts *et al.*, 1985) In 1987, another group of American researchers reported the isolation of HIV from 16 of 66 (24%) haemophiliacs seropositive for HIV [...] (Andrews *et al.*, 1987).
>
> Using the same co-culture techniques and conditions as the above authors, in 1988 Jackson *et al.* tested '75 unselected hemophiliacs ['...] An 'ELISA kit that primarily detects the core p24 antigen of HIV-1' was used to test the culture. [...] They reported HIV isolation from '55 (98%) of 56' haemophiliacs seropositive for HIV and concluded 'that antibody-positive hemophiliacs have been actively infected by HIV-1' (*ibid*, ellipsis and gloss mine)[71]

The Perth Group do not mention Dr Gallo's work in these paragraphs of biomedical literature review and, scouring pp.154-162 of his *Virus Hunters*, I am unable to find the isolation of the 'AIDS virus' that his Index promises. These pages focus on Dr Montagnier and the Institut Louis Pasteur, and the (so far) unsuccessful efforts of Gallo's lab to isolate the virus they were so earnestly hunting for:

> I had already asked [Dr] Marjorie Robert-Guroff [Senior Investigator, Laboratory of Tumor Cell Biology] to check out the AIDS patients' sera carefully for antibodies to HTLVs, even weakly reactive ones. (Gallo/1991/155, gloss mine – from photo caption)[72]

---

[71] The Perth Group use the British spelling of haemophilia and haemophiliac, as is usual in Australia. Full references for these cited papers are provided (Papadopulos-Eleopulos *et al.*/1994b/43-48).

[72] HTLV = Human T-Cell Leukemia Virus, which Dr Gallo (1991/108) admits was "the same type of virus" as ATLV (Adult T-Cell Leukemia Virus) previously

> [Dr] Veffa Franchini [Visiting Scientist, same Lab…] remembers this period from late summer to early fall 1983: "We were still thinking that an HTLV-1 variant […] could be the cause of AIDS […] Marjorie did have 10 percent positivity for HTLV-1 antibodies in patients with AIDS.["] (*ibid*, gloss mine & from photo caption)

> We were surely aware that any retrovirus involved in the cause of AIDS would be substantially different from the known HTLVs. Yet the bulk of evidence, though conflicting and confusing, suggested to me that they would be related. (Gallo/1991/158)

At the end of this chapter Dr Gallo hasn't stated clearly (to my understanding) that HIV was ever isolated. Instead, there is the multiplication of hypotheses, a critique of Dr Montagnier and an admission that the HIV-AIDS link has yet to be proved:

> The only explanation for CC [a cell line][73] was that it contained two viruses: an immortalizing HTLV and the AIDS retrovirus. This in turn led us […] to conclude that Montagnier had been wrong in his statements, made

---

discovered by "[Professor] Yorio Hinuma of Kyoto University", gloss mine. Resolution was similar to that for the conflicting claims of LAV/ HTLV-III. Gallo (*ibid*) also admits that "Japanese investigators, our group, and representatives from England agreed that the virus would be called HTLV, and that the disease would be called ATL, and that more collaboration was imperative." (*ibid*). In 2009, by order of the Japanese government, "Professor Hinuma was conferred with the Order of Culture for the discovery of a retrovirus called the human T-lymphotropic virus type-1 (HTLV-1) which causes adult t-cell leukemia." *Kyoto University*: www.kyoto-u.ac.jp/cutting-edge/awards_honors/research_activities/index6.html – no date, accessed November 2017.

[73] "One of the RT-positive samples would be particularly important to our work. These were the cells from "CC," a Frenchman who had had an accident in Haiti requiring a blood transfusion. Now in Paris, he had been diagnosed as having AIDS." (Gallo/1991/150).

> repeatedly, both in public and in private, that the new kind of retrovirus could not be grown in a cell line. CC was it.
>
> In this new frame of mind, our group headed for the Cold Spring Habor meeting in September 1983. But if our ideas were now firming up, we still did not have laboratory results that clearly linked this new cytopathic [cell-killing], probably LAV-like, retrovirus to the cause of AIDS. (Gallo/1991/161-162, ellipsis & gloss mine & from Index)

The Perth Group, writing three years after the publication of Dr Gallo's book, review more similar literature and comment:

> As can be seen, by HIV isolation is meant detection of one or more of the following phenomena: rarely, virus-like particles and positive hybridization signals for 'viral' RNA, and most often RT and p24. Elsewhere we have presented evidence that detection of these phenomena cannot be considered synonymous with isolation. They can only be used for viral detection if, and only if, they are first shown to be specific to HIV. The above phenomena have been discussed in detail (Papadopulos-Eleopulos, Turner & Papadimitriou, 1993a)[74] and it has been shown that none is specific for HIV or even for retroviruses. (Papadopulos-Eleopulos *et al.*/1994/31)

T-Cells & Viral Load

In their 1992 study, "Latent Viruses and Mutated Oncogenes: No Evidence for Pathogenicity", Professor Duesberg and [Dr] Jody

---

[74] "Is a Positive Western Blot Proof of HIV Infection?". Abstract quoted in full, above, and referenced in text, here, as: (Papadopulos-Eleopulos *et al.*/1993).

R. Schwartz (presumably the researcher listed on a website, updated in 2010, of HIV-AIDS link doubters as "Jody R. Schwartz. PhD" of the Genome Sciences Department, Lawrence Berkeley National Laboratory, Berkeley, California)[75] identify various reasons why HIV cannot be killing T-cells and causing AIDS:

> Since no more than 1 in 500 T-cells of AIDS patients ever contains a DNA provirus of HIV and over 99% of infected T-cells survive infection, and since about 1 in 25 T-cells is regenerated during the 2 days it takes a retrovirus to infect a cell, HIV infection cannot be responsible for the loss of T-cells in AIDS. Thus, HIV, like all other retroviruses, does not kill cells. Indeed, HIV is propagated commercially for the "AIDS test" in cultured lines of the same human T-cells that it is said to kill *in vivo* [in living bodies]. (numbered references omitted, gloss mine)[76]

Two years later, the Perth Group published "A critical analysis of the HIV-T4-cell-AIDS hypothesis", with the following Abstract:

> The data generally accepted as proving the HIV theory of AIDS, HIV cytopathy [cell-killing], destruction of T4 lymphocyctes, and the relationship between T4 cells,

---

[75] www.scribd.com/doc/116726901/Gary-Null-The-Pain-Profit-and-Politics-of-AIDS-Part-1 – posted 2012, accessed November 2017.

[76] Published in *Progress in Nucleic Acid Research and Molecular Biology* 43:135-204, 1992. Available at: www.duesberg.com/papers/ch5.html – posted 1992, accessed November 2017. Dr Jody R. Schwartz is also presumably the same co-author, of the same Genome Sciences Department, of a research paper on human and mouse genomes published by *Genome Research* 11:78-86, in 2001, available on: www.genome.cshlp.org/content/11/1/78.full.pdf – accessed November 2017.

> HIV and the acquired immune deficiency clinical syndrome are critically evaluated. It is concluded these data do not prove that HIV preferentially destroys T4 cells or has any cytopathic effects, nor do they demonstrate that T4 cells are preferentially destroyed in AIDS patients, or that T4 cell destruction and HIV are either necessary or sufficient prerequisites for the development of the clinical syndrome. (Papadopulos-Eleopulos *et al.*/1994a, gloss mine)

Three years later, in 1997, a collaborative paper by [Dr] Mark B. Feinberg and [Professor] Angela R. McLean, then working at the (American) National Institutes of Health and the (French) Institut Pasteur, also questioned the assumptions that CD8 (killer) T-cells play a key role in keeping the HIV 'viral load' down, and that failure of this regulatory mechanism allows HIV to progress to AIDS:

> Two unproven assumptions have stood at the center of the debate about HIV-1 pathogenesis for more than ten years: first, that CTLs [cytotoxic (CD8) T lymphocytes] play the pivotal role in regulating the viral load of an infected individual; second, that the failure of such immune-mediated killing of infected cells is the precipitating event that leads to AIDS. Both of these ideas have been rocked in the last two years. The primacy of immune control of viral load is brought into question by the suggestion that primary viremia [viral load] can terminate in the absence of detectable specific immune responses. Similarly, the suggestion that the failure of immune surveillance is the threshold event that individuals cross as they develop AIDS seems to be inconsistent with data that show no relationship between the rate at which infected individuals clear virus, and the

degree of damage already done to their immune system. (gloss mine, from the same paper)[77]

Which is what Professor Duesberg has been saying all along. HIV has nothing to do with Acquired Immunodeficiency Syndrome:

> The abundance of uninfected T-cells in *all* AIDS patients is the fatal, definitive argument against the many false claims for high viral "loads" or "burdens" in AIDS patients. Nothing could ever stop infectious viruses from infecting all susceptible cells in the same body (except of course antiviral immunity). If T-cells remain uninfected, there are no viruses to infect them. The absence of active, infectious virus automatically disqualifies HIV as a player in the syndrome. (Duesberg & Ellison/1996/176, emphasis original)

Electron Microscopy

In connection with the discovery of RT, Dr Gallo (1991/70) mentions: "we did not have had an electron microscope in the lab". Having shown in 1994 that reverse transcriptase (RT) is not specific to HIV, the Perth Group now took up the topic of this other mode of evidence for the existence of HIV.

> In 2003 the Perth Group emailed Gallo asking if he was aware of the Tahi interview and Montagnier's admission that were no electron micrographs of the BRU [LAV cell line] "purified virus" [...] Gallo replied "Montagnier subsequently published pictures of purified HIV as, of

---

[77] "AIDS: Decline and fall of immune surveillance?" Available at: www.sciencedirect.com/science/article/pii/S0960982297700721 – posted 2004, accessed November 2017.

course, we did in our first papers. You have no need of worry. The evidence is obvious and overwhelming". In fact there was not a single electron micrograph of purified "HIV" published by Gallo in 1984 or since, or by Montagnier. (gloss and ellipsis mine)[78]

The Perth Group quote D. Tahi, interviewing Dr Montagnier and "his electron microscopist colleague and co-author Charles Dauguet", and focus on the lack of evidence for the important claim that (after centrifuge) RT and proteins reacting to antibodies in the BRU serum were seen in a sucrose density gradient of 1.16 g/ml:

> **Tahi**: why do the EM photographs published by you, come from the culture and not from the purification? [the 1.16 g/ml density band]
>
> **Montagnier**: we saw some particles [in the 1.16 g/ml density band] but they did not have the morphology typical of retroviruses. They were very different.
>
> **Tahi**: why no purification?
>
> **Montagnier**: I repeat we did not purify.
>
> **Tahi (to Dauguet)**: How long have you searched in purified gradients before finding the first images of the virus?
>
> **Dauguet**: I first worked on gradients of purified virus for 15 days.
>
> **Tahi**: Have you found viral particles?
>
> **Dauguet**: We have never seen virus particles in the purified virus for 15 days. What we have seen all the

---

[78] P.24, "HIV – A Virus Like No Other", posted 2017, accessed October 2017, available at: http://theperthgroup.com/HIV/TPGVirusLikeNoOther.pdf

time was cellular debris, no virus particles (D. Tahi, personal communication).

Tahi (to Montagnier): Gallo did it [purified]?

Montagnier: Gallo? I don't know if he really purified. I don't believe so. I believe he launched very quickly into the molecular part, that's to say cloning.

Tahi: Today, are the problems about mass production of the virus, purification, EM pictures at 1.16, resolved?

Montagnier: Yes. of course.

Tahi: Do EM pictures of HIV from the purification exist?

Montagnier: Yes. of course.

Tahi: Have they been published?

Montagnier: I couldn't tell you...we have somewhere...but it is not of interest...not of any interest.

In other words, Montagnier and his colleagues had a purified 1.16 g/ml band, but what they purified was cellular debris, not retrovirus particles. Nonetheless, they called the 1.16 g/ml band "purified, labeled virus".[79]

Dr Ben Goldacre (2009/182) states that "AIDS is the opposite of anecdote." Tragically, for all those already maimed and killed over more than thirty years by an unproven but exceedingly lucrative hypothesis, it appears that, still, the evidence for the harmful effects of HIV – or even for its existence – may be nothing more than circumstantial and anecdotal.

---

[79] Gloss, bold emphasis and ellipsis original. The interview is referenced by footnote as: "at the Pasteur Institute July 18th 1997. *Continuum* 1998. 5:30-34." Perth Group, *op. cit.*, p.21.

Deaths of Dissidents

One of the more distasteful activities of (some) AIDS activists is celebrating the deaths of AIDS dissidents, sometimes irrespective of whether or not the reported cause is on the current CDC list of over twenty opportunistic infections (see below). 'Celebrating' is, disgracefully, not too strong a word. 'Sneering' may also aptly describe the attitude of a blogger with the pseudonym "Phrost" of the blogpost, "That Time When an AIDS Conspiracy Magazine Went Out of Business Because the Employees Died of AIDS", which features a photo of three healthy-looking young people pointing and laughing.[80] The employees mentioned are the editors of the above-mentioned, professionally-written, *Continuum* magazine, which (at least in the articles I've read) focussed on uncensored scientific discussion not conspiracy theories.

Dr Kendrick (2014/33) reminds us that "we're all going to die" and that "one form of life-saving can clearly be of much greater value than the other" (2014/34). In the case of AIDS dissidents who have previously been on various drugs including AZT and who then stop taking (at least some of) them and die decades later, the relevant response surely is not to wonder at (or celebrate) their demise but to be grateful that they had more time alive than their more docile peers

---

[80] Available at: www.bullshido.net/that-time-when-an-aids-conspiracy-magazine-went-out-of-business-because-the-employees-died-of-aids/ – no date, accessed November 2017.

who on medical instruction kept taking the tablets and lived only a few years after they started to do so. There is the added complication that some dissidents are persuaded (not to say bullied) by well-meaning friends and family to resubmit themselves to the antiretroviral regime and their demise shortly follows. The late Christine Maggiore is such an example.

Human nature being what it is, the deaths of these celebrated people attract much attention and if Professor Duesberg or a member of the Perth Group should ever come down with "**Candidiasis of bronchi, trachea, esophagus, or lungs**" or "**Invasive cervical cancer**" or "**Coccidioidomycosis**" or "**Cryptococcosis**" or "**Cryptosporidiosis, chronic intestinal (greater than one month's duration)**" or "**Cytomegalovirus diseases (particularly retinitis) (CMV)**" or "**Encephalopathy, HIV-related**" or "**Herpes simplex (HSV): chronic ulcer(s) (greater than one month's duration); or bronchitis, pneumonitis, or esophagitis**" or "**Histoplasmosis**" or "**Isosporiasis, chronic intestinal (greater than one month's duration)**" or "**Kaposi's sarcoma (KS)**" or "**Lymphoma, multiple forms**" or "**Tuberculosis (TB)**" or "***Mycobacterium* avium complex (MAC) or *Mycobacterium kansasii*, disseminated or extrapulmonary. Other *Mycobacterium*, disseminated or extrapulmonary.**" Or "***Pneumocystis carinii* pneumonia (PCP)**" or "**Pneumonia, recurrent**" or "**Progressive multifocal leukoencephalopathy**" or "*Salmonella* **septicemia, recurrent**" or "**Toxoplasmosis of brain**" or "**Wasting syndrome due to HIV**",[81] after decades of health rather than dying of liver failure a few years after starting HAART, we can expect similar sneers.

One of the many problems with anecdotal evidence is that there are always opposing anecdotes. Professor Duesberg (1996/348-359) relates, compassionately, "the stories of those who believed in AZT" (all caps in original) among them Kimberly Bergalis who was apparently a healthy nineteen year-old until she started taking AZT and survived for two painful years; Alison Gertz who was apparently a healthy twenty-two year-old until she started taking AZT, and survived for four; and Wimbledon champion Arthur Ashe who, after a heart attack at the age of thirty-six, was pronounced HIV positive and whose health plummeted on AZT for the five years till his death.

Each complained of the effects of their treatment:

> I have lived through the torturous ache that infested my face and neck, brought on by AZT. I have endured trips twice a week to Miami for three months only to receive painful IV injections. I've had blood transfusions. I've had a bone marrow biopsy. I cried my heart out from the pain. (Kimberly Bergalis, quoted in Duesberg & Ellison/1996/350)

> [Alison] Gertz started AZT treatment in 1989. The 1990 *People* magazine profile recounted the consequent disaster: (Duesberg & Ellison/1996/354, gloss mine)

> Last October she was hospitalized with a severe allergic reaction to AZT. When the doctors called for a lung biopsy, Ali balked. "I told them if they were going to put

---

[81] www.cdc.gov/hiv/basics/livingwithhiv/opportunisticinfections.html – updated 30th May 2017, accessed 29th November 2017. Bold emphasis and italics original.

me to sleep, I'd never wake up," she says. "My strength was gone." Released after 17 days, she recuperated at home, where her mother and girlfriends took turns nursing her around the clock. "They'd help me to the bathroom, feed me, see that I didn't fall in the shower," says Ali. "My knees were so bony I had to sleep with a pillow between them." (*People*, quoted *ibid*)

Just as soon as [Arthur] Ashe received his AIDS diagnosis in 1988, his doctor pushed him into taking AZT. He started on an unbelievably high dose, nearly double the seriously toxic levels used in the Phase II trial. His doctor only gradually lowered the dose over the next four years. "I refuse to dwell on how much damage I may have done to myself taking the higher dosage," Ashe later admitted. (Duesberg & Ellison/1996/357, gloss mine)

It was symptoms such as these which led Christine Maggiore, founder of the HIV diagnosis survivors' website www.aliveandwell, to seek for alternative answers to the cause of her condition. Diagnosed in 1992, she similarly suffered on AZT but made the decision (until finally pressured otherwise) to stay off antiretrovirals and survived not for two, four or five years but for eighteen.

ART & Liver Failure

Anecdotal evidence is fundamentally flawed, especially when reported by the unqualified in sneering online articles lacking as much in human compassion as in journalistic integrity. When evidence is gathered with a transparent and appropriate methodology by experts in the field who are unafraid of the honest presentation of data, then it carries weight.

Commenting on the need to correct figures for the ever-growing multitude of official "AIDS-defining diseases" with those for their "normal occurrence" in "HIV-free controls", Professor Duesberg (1996/425) sums up his argument:

> There is no evidence that HIV-positive people who are not drug users have a higher morbidity or mortality than HIV-free controls.
>
> David Ho, director of the Aaron Diamond AIDS Research Centre of New York, recently gave the key to long-term survival with HIV: "None had received antiretroviral therapy."[82]

In case this conclusion is dismissed as out-of-date, even "Human immunodeficiency virus and liver disease: A comprehensive update", a study last month (November 2017) clearly links ART to liver failure. Perhaps not *clearly*. The sponsorship by several large pharmaceutical companies negates that possibility, despite official denial:

> Potential conflict of interest: Dr. Sherman [Gould Professor of Medicine, Director of Division of Digestive Diseases at the University of Cincinnati] received grants through his institution from AbbVie, BMS, Gilead,

---

[82] Professor Duesberg references this study in an endnote as: "Y. Cao, L. Quin, L. Zhang, J. Safrit, and D.D. Ho, "Virologic and Immunologic Characterization of Long-Term Survivors of Human Immunodificiency Virus Type 1 Infection," *New England Journal of Medicine*, 332 (1995): 201-208."

Innovio, Intercept, MedImmune, and Merck; he is also an advisor to Gilead, Merck, and MedImmune and is on the Data and Safety Monitoring Board for MedPace and Watermark. The other authors declare no conflict of interest.[83]

Lest we imagine that the other authors (Dr Marion G. Peters, Professor of Medicine at UCSF and Chief of Hepatology [liver] Research; and Dr David Lee Thomas, Professor of Medicine and Director of the Division of Infectious Diseases at John Hopkins University) are free from pressure to published 'big pharma'-friendly results, I note who funded the conference that this paper was, presumably, presented at – and remember that any researcher who does not follow the party line is denied such a platform:

> Supported by educational grants from Gilead Sciences, Inc.; Janssen Therapeutics, Division of Janssen Products; Merck & Co.; ViiV Healthcare; Intercept Pharmaceuticals, Inc.; and Tobira Therapeutics, Inc. Funding for this conference was made possible in part by the National Institutes of Health under Award Number R13AI071925 to K.E.S. from the National Institute of Allergy and Infectious Diseases, with cofunding from the National Institute on Drug Abuse.[84]

Nevertheless, the Introduction reveals a significant lack of communication in medical care:

---

[83] *Hepatology Communications*, Vol. 1 Issue 10, December 2017, pp. 987-1001. Available at: http://onlinelibrary.wiley.com/doi/10.1002/hep4.1112/full – published online 6th November 2017, accessed 6th December 2017. Gloss mine.

[84] *Ibid.*

Although increased numbers of HIV care providers have embraced provision of newer direct-acting antiviral (DAA) HCV [Hepatitis C Virus] therapies, the linkage between hepatologists and those managing individuals infected with HIV remains limited in most places.[85]

Disturbing enough, but the chart below the Introduction reveals a steep curve of "Clinical liver-related complications", rising from a baseline in 1990 – three years after AZT was licensed for HIV – to a peak at the end of reported data, in 2013 (the chart, bizarrely, imagining a downturn, continues on to 2030) which dwarfs the curves of complications in both drug-induced liver injury and intravenous drug users. The erudite authors of this heavily-pharma-funded paper, have this, very tentative, backwardly-stated conclusion, that ART=death:

> The extent to which ART [antiretroviral therapy] *attenuates* these mechanisms is difficult to determine; however, clinical studies reveal residual increased risk of liver fibrosis progression *even* among those taking ART.[86]

---

[85] *Ibid.* Gloss from "Abbreviations" glossary.

[86] *Ibid.* Gloss and emphasis mine.

AFTERWORD & *APOLOGIA*

This short book is, and can only be, a very inadequate summary of certain aspects (hopefully the principle aspects) of the hypotheses of AIDS that have been publically debated since 1984 and have their roots in research from years before the declaration to the press that 'HIV is the probable cause of AIDS'. I hope it will serve as a fairly adequate signpost to the published work of those who have formulated these conflicting, and sometime overlapping, hypotheses – especially now that some of this work has fallen under the ban of 'no-platforming'.

I repeat that I am unqualified to have an opinion on this theoretical conflict, at least an opinion that anyone should be swayed by. I reserve the right to have a personal viewpoint and that is, now: at the end of these intensive months of reading (one can hardly call it 'study') which follow years of sporadic interest in the subject, I am not much further forward. I am about 99% sure that this HIV-AIDS link has never been proved to be factual. I can confidently say, at least, that it has never been proved to my satisfaction.

I am unqualified in biomedical matters, but I am not unqualified in philosophy. Although my doctoral thesis applied my metaphysical (ontological) research to the field of education, the discipline named 'the love of wisdom' is one: my original inspiration was in mechanics, specifically motorcycle maintenance, and my thesis contained many reflections on the philosophy of science, especially those of the incomparable moral philosopher and opponent of the categorical confusions of scientism, Mary Midgley, twice honoured with a doctorate and retired Senior Lecturer at the University of Newcastle.

My doctoral research also focussed on paradigm change and I was particularly struck by the qualification of the Scottish philosopher of science, Professor Alasdair Chalmers MacIntyre (1974), of the University of Notre Dame (and of other US and UK universities), to the work of the American Professor (at Berkeley, Princeton & MIT) Thomas Samuel Kuhn (1962) on the subject: Professor Kuhn sees, in the succession of philosophical paradigms, the human tendency to construct narrative flow. However, Professor MacIntyre points out that paradigm shift occurs more often in epistemological crisis (crises of knowledge) than in continuity.

Although this book has largely presented scientific criticism of the work of Dr Robert Gallo, I must say that I enjoyed reading his *Virus Hunting* immensely – precisely because of the narrative flow. Nevertheless, I take Professor MacIntyre's point about a crisis of knowledge and Professor Kuhn's about revolutions in thought. So does Professor Bauer:

> Mainstream science sticks to theories that had once been accepted by ignoring anomalies, conundrums, absurdities for as long as possible (Thomas S. Kuhn [...]). Things that don't fit an existing theory are accommodated by *ad hoc* adjustments (Imre Lakatos [...]), just as Ptolemy long maintained belief in the circular perfection of

heavenly motions by adding epicycles upon epicycles, wheels within wheels, to avoid acknowledging that the movements are not really circular after all.

So too HIV/AIDS researchers create new hypotheses to bolster their belief whenever they seem unable to explain what they observe. Since all the data point to HIV not being infective, or being apparently infective to so low a degree as to be incapable of producing an epidemic, auxiliary hypotheses were suggested which have become accepted as shibboleths:

1. The epidemic in Africa is said to have come about because of an incredible rate of promiscuity. Sexually active South Africans (black South Africans, that is) are postulated to have an average of 10 sexual partners at any give[n] time and to change them about annually (pp. 63-65 in James Chin, *The AIDS Pandemic*, Radcliffe 2007).

2. Soon after initial infection, there is an "acute phase" where large amounts of HIV are present, and intercourse during that phase makes transmission much more likely: infectivity is very high during these short periods, so overall measurements of transmissibility are deceiving.

The first suggestion is absurd, since such behavior would be so visibly evident that it could not be overlooked; yet it is not observed.

The second suggestion has been undermined by a careful re-analysis of the single study on which it had been based: the "excess hazard-months attributable to the acute phase of infection" is about 5.3, not the previously estimated 31-to-141 (Bellan et al., "Reassessment of HIV-1 acute phase infectivity: accounting for heterogeneity and study design with simulated cohorts", *PLoS Medicine*, 12(3): e1001801).[87]

To paraphrase Dr Gallo, the evidence for this belief may be overwhelming – in terms of the proliferation of published studies on the subject – but it's by no means obvious. Especially as the official story is as complicated as this:

HIV – that's the multiple groups and subtypes of HIV-1 and HIV-2 – came from Africa, having mutated from some harmless monkey disease (no-one is exactly sure which monkey) some time in the last 3 million years. This mutation definitely had nothing to do with the widespread monkey virus contamination of human cell lines reported in laboratories worldwide. After not mutating for perhaps millions of years, HIV has done nothing but mutate since the 70s. This makes sense. By a combination of means (including prostitution, package holidays, cannibalism and voodoo) HIV turned up in the blood cells of a French gentleman who had been holidaying in Haiti.

This virus – which may or may not be exactly the same reported to be stolen by the American who patented it for his lucrative HIV test – was said to be isolated at the time of discovery even though later on the French discoverer admitted that it really wasn't. Fortunately, someone invented something called PCR that can make viral haystacks out of needles – and even though he

---

[87] https://hivskeptic.wordpress.com/category/mf-ratios/ – published online 31st July 2016, accessed 7th December 2017. Ellipsis & gloss mine. Lakatos referenced as: "Imre Lakatos ("History of science and its rational reconstruction", pp. 1-40 in *Method and Appraisal in the Physical Sciences*, ed. Colin Howson, Cambridge University Press 1976)".

explicitly says that this can't be done for HIV we have no need to believe him because apparently he once took LSD.

The American then was apparently pressurised into having it announced as the probable cause of AIDS (and pressurised into patenting it for roughly US$17 million) but the press dropped the 'probable' the next day and scientists followed suit. Also dropped at this time were any alternative explanations for the collection of diseases some of which (but not all, including the most iconic) were connected to failure of the immune system. This collection, now to be known as ARC, manifested especially in drug-users. But this fact has to be completely ignored as it's incidental. As is the almost universal use of alkyl nitrates by gay men.

Fortunately the CDC just happened to have a wee drug handy. The fact that it had been found to be too toxic for human use and that those that took it now died sooner than those that didn't is neither here nor there. What we need to believe is that it was the best thing available at the time – and had absolutely nothing to do with the huge amounts of money made by its manufacturers. The fact that the same manufacturers have massively supported AIDS events which encourage people to get tested and to start on the drugs as soon as possible is, again, neither here nor there. It just shows that some people have big hearts, obviously.

The patented test was to protect the blood supply and the huge number of false positives its faulty parameters produced is in no way evidence for the fear and loathing that White heterosexual

Americans had in the 1980's for Black people, gay men and drug users. Similarly, the fact that the patented test was not to be used for diagnosis of 'HIV positive' individuals and it was, massively, is again absolutely no fault of the manufacturers – who included a wee note to that effect and so are entirely blameless (this whole story is one of selfless sanctity all round).

Now that over thirty years have passed and the opposition has (mostly) been shouted down, we can only shed a tear of regret over the unfortunate deaths from AZT earlier. Now, however, we need to look on the bright side and get on with getting everyone, absolutely everyone, tested as soon as possible (even the babies, especially the babies) and getting everyone possible on anti-HIV drugs. In case anyone feels left out, there's always PEP to take after coming into contact with any bodily fluid whatsoever, and PrEP to take if you haven't already but feel you might, at some point. So, really, we can all get on them. This, again, isn't for large pharmaceutical companies to make money, Heaven forbid! No! It's just to be on the safe side. It's for our own good. We'll also just ignore the rise tide of death by liver failure. That, obviously, has absolutely nothing to do with antiretrovirals which are 100% safe! Well, not 100% but then nothing is and, in fact, the large pharmaceutical companies that make them are 100% not liable for any side effects because they're all (and there are quite a few of them) listed on the wee bit of paper inside the box.

Meanwhile, the number of White, heterosexual, females with HIV is rising. This has absolutely nothing to do with the insistence that absolutely everyone should get tested. Also, the criminalisation of seropositive sex is only just, the multiplicity of strains is evidence, and large-scale quarantine will only be used when necessary.

A complicated story indeed! Still, I can't be 100% sure. It shouldn't matter to the reader if I were. I am unqualified and anyone who takes a medical decision based on my perceived opinion is a fool. What I am even more convinced about is that over thirty years of treating Professor Duesberg, Dr Mullis and the Perth Group as dangerous heretics is not only unjust to them personally and professionally but also has impoverished the debate over these hypotheses to the point where the established order may be described, without much exaggeration, as inquisitorial.

At the end of this book, I wish to add a personal note. I have many friends whose involvement with these hypotheses is far from theoretical. Would that it were. Some of these friends have died. Some work in the caring industry and some are educators. Some are volunteers for various charitable organisations. Some fundraise. Some are currently taking anti-HIV drugs.

I am aware that my writing this book may seem – to at least some of these friends – to be (at best) an impertinence and (at worst) a betrayal. Some may even feel that it constitutes a reckless endangerment of lives. They may be right. In my defence, I can only point out the competent authorities whose words I have tried to publish, again, so that more people may listen to them; I can only testify to what I have learned of their academic and professional character, setting out as evidence of the authenticity of their motivations the fact that their careers would surely have benefitted had they kept to the party line. I can only remind readers that, on the other side, there are cases of error and fraud which are a matter of public record, some of which I have alluded to in passing.

Even should the tide of public opinion turn and AIDS be recognised as an incoherent set of unrelated diseases, and HIV as either a harmless passenger virus or as an empirical error over protein particles in cellular debris, let us not hunt the virus hunters.

Let us, instead, persistently question authority and hold it accountable; let us not allow our desperation for miracle cures for the sick to lead us into destruction of the healthy; let us embrace the embarrassment and discomfort that accompanies admitting error openly on the path of truth; and let us mourn the innocence of all our beloved dead, and comfort those whom healers have so grievously afflicted.

BIBLIOGRAPHY

Bennett, Rebecca and Erin, Charles, A. (2001) *HIV and AIDS: Testing, Screening, and Confidentiality*. New York: Oxford University Press.

Blair, E.; Darby, G.; Gough, G.; Littler, E.; Rowlands, D.; and Tisdale, M. (1998) *Antiviral Therapy*. Oxford: Bios Scientific Publishers.

Corbitt, Gerald (2001) "HIV Testing and Screening: Current Practicalities and Future Possibilities", in Bennett and Erin (2001) pp.21-38.

Craddock, Mark (2006) "Some mathematical considerations on HIV and AIDS", in Duesberg (1996) pp.89-95.

Davis, Steven (2010) *Are You Positive?* Ibiza, Spain: L&G Productions.

Duesberg, Peter H. (1994) "Foreign-protein-mediated immunodeficiency in hemophiliacs with and without HIV", in Duesberg (1996) pp.49-68.

Duesberg, Peter H. (Ed.) (1996) *Aids: Virus- or Drug Induced?* Contemporary Issues in Genetics and Evolution, Volume 5. Boston (MASS.): Kluwer Academic Publishers.

Duesberg, Peter H. and Ellison, Bryan J. (1996) *Inventing the Aids Virus*. Washington (DC): Regnery Publishing.

Duh, Samuel V. (1991) *Blacks and Aids: Causes and Origins*. Sage Series on Race and Ethnic Relations Vol. 3. London: Sage Publications.

Farber Celia (1996) "The HIV test", in Duesberg (1996) pp.343-358.

Feldman, Douglas A. and Wang Miller, Julia (Eds) (1998) *The AIDS Crisis: A Documentary History*. London: Greenwood Press.

Gallo, Robert (1991) *Virus Hunting: AIDS, Cancer and the Human Retrovirus: A Story of Scientific Discovery*. New York (NY): BasicBooks (HarperCollins).

Gelderblom, Hans R.; Marx, Preston A.; Özel Muhsin; Gheysen, Dirk; Munn, Robert J.; Joy, Kenneth I. and Pauli, Georg (1990) "Morphogenesis, Maturation and Fine Structure of Lentiviruses", in Pearl (1990) pp.159-180.

Goldacre, Ben (2009) *Bad Science*. London: Fourth Estate.

Goldacre, Ben (2012) *Bad Pharma: How drug companies mislead doctors and harm patients*. London: Fourth Estate.

Harris, Steven B. (1996) "AIDS and good theory-making", in Duesberg (1996) pp.231-239.

Hodgkinson, Neville (1996) "Cry, beloved country: How Africa became the victim of a non-existent epidemic of HIV/AIDS", in Duesberg (1996) pp.347-358.

Johnson, Philip E. (1996) "The Thinking Problem in HIV-science", in Duesberg (1996) pp.331-336.

Jones, Steve and Van Loon, Borin (2001) *Introducing Genetics*. Cambridge (UK): Icon Books.

Kendrick, Dr Malcolm (2014) *Doctoring Data: How to sort out medical advice from medical nonsense*. Cwmbran, Wales: Columbus.

Kuhn, Thomas (1962) *The Structure of Scientific Revolutions*. Chicago: University of Chicago Press.

MacIntyre, Alasdair (1974) "Epistemological Crises, Dramatic Narrative, and the Philosophy of Science" in Joyce Oldham Appleby (Ed.) (1996) *Knowledge and Postmodernism in Historical Perspective*. London: Routledge, pp.357-367.

McManus, Alan (2011) *Alchemy at the Chalkface: Pirsig, Pedagogy and the Metaphysics of Quality*. Glasgow: Alan McManus.

McManus, Alan (2013) *Only Say The Word: Affirming Gay and Lesbian Love*. Alresford, Hants (UK): Christian Alternative.

McManus, Alan (2015) *Life Choice: the Ethics and Ideologies of Abortion*. Glasgow: Alan McManus.

McManus, Alan (2016) *'Time for Inclusive Education' and the Conservative Catholic*. Glasgow: Alan McManus.

McManus, Alan (2017) *Trans/Substantiation: The Metaphysics of Transgender*. Glasgow: Alan McManus.

Papadopulos-Eleopulos, E; Turner, V.F.; Papadimitrou, J.M. (1993) "Is a Positive Western Blot Proof of HIV Infection?", *Bio/Technology*, Vol. 11, pp.696-707.

Papadopulos-Eleopulos, E; Turner, Valendar. F.; Papadimitrou, John M.; Causer, David; Hedland-Thomas, Bruce; Page, Barry A.P. (1994a) "A critical analysis of the HIV-T4-cell-AIDS hypothesis", in Duesberg (1996) pp.3-22.

Papadopulos-Eleopulos, E; Turner, V.F.; Papadimitrou, J.M.; Causer, D. (1994b) "Factor VIII, HIV and AIDS in haemophiliacs: an analysis of their relationship", in Duesberg (1996) pp.23-48.

Pearl, Laurence, H. (Ed.) (1990) *Retroviral Proteases: control of maturation and morphogenesis*. London: Macmillan.

Root-Bernstein, Robert S. (1994) "Five myths about AIDS that have misdirected research and treatment", in Duesberg (1996) pp.185-206.

Stewart, Gordon T. (1994) "The epidemiology and transmission of AIDS: a hypothesis linking behavioural and biological determinants to time, person and place", in Duesberg (1996) pp.163-183.

ABOUT THE AUTHOR

Alan McManus, M.Theol. (hons), M.Phil, PGDE, M.Litt., Ph.D., is a freelance academic, novelist, playwright and dramaturg. His doctoral thesis, *Alchemy at the Chalkface: Pirsig, Pedagogy and the Metaphysics of Quality*, is on the work of the creative and contrarian American Philosopher, Dr Robert M. Pirsig.

Only Say The Word: Affirming Gay and Lesbian Love, (Christian Alternative, 2013) is the first, *Life-Choice: the Ethics and Ideologies of Abortion* the second, and *Trans/Substantiation: The Metaphysics of Transgender* the third, in a series of books based on his doctoral thesis. This thesis and his ethnographic dissertation, *Dreaming Anarchy: a Shut-Eye View of a Utopia*, are discussed in his chapter, "Strange Attractors: Myth, Dream, and Memory in Educational Methodology", in the *International Handbook of Interpretation in Educational Research* (Springer, 2015). He has also published articles on political philosophy and WW1 remembrance in the online journal, *Citizenship, Social and Economics Education*.

DEAR READER

Thank-you for reading this book. Please consider reviewing *Silence & Dissent* on your favourite online retailer and telling your friends about it in person and via social media. You can let me know about reviews through Twitter: @gumptionology

Alan

www.ingramcontent.com/pod-product-compliance
Lightning Source LLC
Chambersburg PA
CBHW020436220526
45464CB00002B/736